The Zimmer, The Hat and The Collie: Looking for Alan

I0090100

by
Issy Burrows

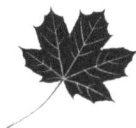

MAPLE
PUBLISHERS

The Zimmer, The Hat and The Collie: Looking for Alan

Author: Issy Burrows

Copyright © 2024 Issy Burrows

The right of Issy Burrows to be identified as author of this work has been asserted by the author in accordance with section 77 and 78 of the Copyright, Designs and Patents Act 1988.

ISBN 978-1-83538-398-8 (Paperback)
      978-1-83538-399-5 (Hardback)
      978-1-83538-400-8 (E-Book)

Book Cover Design and Layout by:
      White Magic Studios
      www.whitemagicstudios.co.uk

Published by:
      Maple Publishers
      Fairbourne Drive, Atterbury,
      Milton Keynes,
      MK10 9RG, UK
      www.maplepublishers.com

Acknowledgements

My heartfelt thanks go to Maple Publishing, with special appreciation for Pam, who expertly guided me through every step of the process. I am grateful to the proofreading team for boosting my confidence in my script, and to the illustrator for capturing the light-hearted spirit I envisioned for the book cover.

I am especially thankful for Mum's dedicated carers, whose exceptional care allowed her to remain comfortably at home while I was at work. Their kindness and commitment brought comfort and joy to her daily life.

To my family, thank you for your unwavering support, especially Ashley and Cameron, whose encouragement inspired me to write this book. My deepest gratitude goes to my dear husband, Andrew, for his endless support throughout this journey, and for his boundless kindness and respect for Mum during her time with us.

CONTENTS

Preface

This book is a collection of memories of my experience of living with someone who has been diagnosed with Alzheimer's dementia and how a family adapts, learns to cope and bond together in the face of challenging behaviour. The book highlights how emotional intelligence and going with the flow can work in the favour of the carer when caring for a relative with dementia.

My first experience of knowing someone with Alzheimer's was when I was a twelve year old child and my Grandmother came to live with us. This book includes black humour as part of the observations of knowing someone or living with someone with dementia through the eyes of a child and later on as an adult. When I was eighteen I commenced my nurse training and qualified as a registered nurse at the age of twenty-one. During my nursing career I have had a vast experience of caring for elderly people with dementia. I worked in an elderly care hospital as my first post following registration. Throughout my career I have gained valuable experience with dementia patients in any setting and I have also been a matron of a nursing home. I have also had further experience recently when I cared for my Mother during the Covid pandemic, who also had been diagnosed with Alzheimer's. Managing our own occupational health business and dealing with the Covid pandemic added layers of complexities whilst caring for Mum. Caring for a relative with dementia is challenging and can be taken on as a responsibility but in my opinion only love will see you through this.

This book is about life and death. It's about the hidden struggles that people encounter when caring for a relative with dementia. It's a book that delves into the depths of despair but it's also a book of laughter and reflection. This is not meant to be a miserable book even though it touches on grief and profound difficulties and at times anguish. There are many precious memories and funny stories that a stand-up comedian would relish. The story is a true one and it is not always politically correct but it is real. It captures the realities of a family learning together how best to adapt to cope with living with a relative who has dementia. It also points out that sometimes it goes badly wrong. The family learns by trial and error and there is no training or education available so you just muddle along.

It is also a story of contrast, of how a loved one dying at home can be, in a strange way gratifying, whereas a loved one dying where any control has been taken away and communication fails can lead to long lasting consequences for the relatives left behind. I chose to write this book for three reasons; the first was to hopefully assist me with the grief process, the second reason was for education purposes as I believe people need to understand more about the realities of caring for a relative with Alzheimer's in their own home and the third reason was to reassure people in a similar situation that they are not alone. I have always loved caring for elderly people so it came naturally to me to want to care for my family. I am also a qualified nurse and I understand the system better than most but even to me some of the politics around care, I find baffling. It was through my experiences as well as my professional background that I felt I had something to give other people by writing about my experiences. As I started to write the book it took on a life of its own and set off in different directions than I was expecting it to go. The story also touches on some local dialect and social cultures. Animals have always been a big part of our family life and I couldn't write this book without including our beloved animal friends.

Leisure by William Henry Davies

What is this life if, full of care,
We have no time to stand and stare?—

No time to stand beneath the boughs,
And stare as long as sheep and cows:

No time to see, when woods we pass,
Where squirrels hide their nuts in grass:

No time to see, in broad daylight,
Streams full of stars, like skies at night:

No time to turn at Beauty's glance,
And watch her feet, how they can dance:

No time to wait till her mouth can
Enrich that smile her eyes began?

A poor life this if, full of care,
We have no time to stand and stare.

The poem above was a favourite of my Dad and was recited by my husband, at his funeral.

The book is mainly about Sybil Boote (my Mum), Alan Boote (my Dad) and Grandma Beech (my Mum's, Mum). If I had to describe them collectively, they were modest and humble people who knew the true value of life. They were honest, they didn't dress things up to placate, they called a spade a spade.

Chapter 1

On Reflection

When I think back, there were signs that Mum had started with Dementia long before we suspected it and many years before it was diagnosed. One example of what I now suspect was a sign that I can recall is when myself and my husband Andrew had gone around to visit Mum and Dad at their house in Eaton Road in Alsager. Their house was a modest semi-detached one in a pleasant and friendly neighbourhood of the town. Alsager used to be a village but it has grown over the years and was now classed as a town but it retained its village feel and community spirit and many people knew each other.

In the front room of their house, there were two large settees covered in Mum's crocheted blankets. The settees were positioned at right angles to each other. Mum was sitting on one of the settees and Dad was sitting on the other. Both of my parents were fairly technophobic, however, Dad liked to have a mobile phone. He had just bought himself a new 'Pay as You Go' mobile phone. When he was a young man he was a keen cyclist and he had taken this hobby up again when he was sixty-eight years old until a couple of years before his death. He cycled about twenty five miles every other day and he was very fit, regularly cycling with Andrew and myself. He rose to the challenge of completing many charity cycles with us across the beautiful spellbinding Scottish islands such as Aaron and Mull as well as the mainland of the west coast of Scotland.

He carried a mobile phone when he went out cycling just in case of emergencies. Dad had lots of trouble using it though because the buttons were so small, he would often hit the wrong numbers. His hands were gigantic worker's hands, his fingers were chubby like Cumberland sausages and they seemed clumsy. On this particular day, Dad wanted to try out his new mobile phone to make sure he was using it correctly. He informed Mum that he would phone her on the landline to check that his new mobile phone was working. He clumsily keyed in the home landline telephone number with his chubby fingers and the landline phone began to ring. Mum picked up the receiver to answer the call.

'Hello,' she said in her best telephone voice.

'Hello, it's me.'

'Who is this please?' she said in a stern voice.

'It's me, Alan.'

'Oh, I have a husband called Alan.'

'It's me, you silly bugger,' Dad replied into the phone, waving and pointing to the phone from the other settee.

Andrew and I watched this hilarious sketch in disbelief, I had tears rolling down my face and couldn't stop laughing. Afterwards, we remarked that Peter Kay could do a lot with the sketch that we had just witnessed. Looking back at this moment, I now wonder whether this was one of the first signs that Mum was getting confused and could not comprehend what Dad was doing. Maybe this was the first sign of dementia.

It is important to note at this point that Mum and Dad were never very PC, that is politically correct, whilst at the same time being the most forgiving, accepting and non-judgemental couple you could wish to meet. They would often swear at each other but with no malice. In a strange way swearing at each other was a form of affection. Mum never used really naughty words though, but she would quite comfortably say 'Silly Bugger' or 'Arseholes'. Dad also used these terminologies, but he had been known in extreme circumstances though never in front of Mum to use the F word. However, 'Silly Bugger' was an endearing term for both of them whereas 'Arseholes' was definitely not.

There were other signs of early onset dementia too but Mum became an expert in covering up. She became an enthusiastic user of sticky 'Post It' notes as well as writing messages, birthdays and other notes on pieces of paper. She was never wasteful and would use ripped up pieces of paper from used envelopes or she would use the cardboard to write on out of a new pair of tights. She started to cover these pieces of paper and cardboard with messages or telephone numbers. She would write shopping lists of things that she wanted to buy which is quite normal and so I never thought anything of it until I would find another identical list and then another. I am a big fan of lists too. However, there was a ridiculous amount of pieces of paper with telephone numbers, birthday dates and written lists. I would find duplicates of sticky notes with mine, Andrew's and Allister's (my brother) telephone number written on. As the dementia progressed, more and more sticky notes appeared. This was less obvious when Dad was alive; with the same routine and familiar surrounding she managed to hide the subtle signs. Dad was Mum's rock, compass and settling influence. He kept her in check when she became a bit naughty. He was the car driver in the family and the person that took care of the DIY in the house and garden. My parents were keen gardeners and both took pride in their home. And they had a busy social life, were very popular and they did everything together. They had always put great importance on family. Allister's and my memories from childhood are very precious. Mum and Dad were great role models and we were a tight knit family.

In June 2014, Dad told me that he had been experiencing some unpleasant symptoms when he went to the toilet and after ignoring them for a while he eventually went to see his doctor. He was referred to the hospital for a routine scope. I drove Dad to the hospital with Mum as they had told him not to drive. Mum and I waited in the area designated for waiting relatives. I had no reason to be concerned as these types of tests are often routine, so Mum and I sat there relaxed and chatting away. A nurse came out of the clinical area and asked for Mrs Boote to come through to her husband and the doctor.

'I will go and fetch him Mum, you wait here.'

'No, we need Mrs Boote to come through.'

'Can I come too?'

'Yes, I'm sure that is fine.'

I could tell something was very wrong and I felt my legs go weak. Mum was oblivious. The doctor was my parents' GP and a family friend and he gently broke the news that Dad had bowel cancer. Dad needed surgery to remove part of his colon and then further scans to see if the cancer had spread to other parts of his body. This cancer diagnosis was devastating news and we as a family climbed on board the roller coaster of cancer treatment. We had despair one minute and hope the next. The following two and a half years entailed surgery, chemotherapy and other experimental treatments. On occasions, there was hope of a cure but this was short lived as we were told that the cancer had spread to his lymph nodes, lungs and liver. There was a discussion about removing part of his liver and treating the lung cancer with radiotherapy. I drove Mum and Dad down to the Queen Elizabeth hospital in Birmingham to see a liver specialist. The specialist doctor sat behind a desk with his feet and shoes resting on the desk, swinging from side to side. He then sat up and bluntly told my father that if they operated he would not survive the operation because too much liver would have to be removed and it would kill him. I think that the doctor had not learnt bedside manners and it was quite shocking how he behaved. There is no nice way to deliver such news but this blunt delivery was shocking. My Dad, this hard man, this caring man, this very intelligent man, this rock, came out of the hospital shaking with fear and he couldn't believe how the doctor had his feet on the desk and was so casual about dashing Dad's hopes. The doctor had come to this conclusion just from looking at the scans which surely he could have done without us making the two hour journey to get there. He could have contacted Dad's oncologist or he could have telephoned his GP and saved us time that now was not a given but a luxury. I remember the journey home from Birmingham, there was a strange, deafening and awkward silence that was alien to our family. There were no words of comfort or optimism, just anguish and distress.

Then came hope to visit again as there was some experimental treatment on offer. This experimental treatment was to block off the liver and fill it with chemotherapy. The liver would be blocked off so that the poison could not escape and move to other vital organs. Even though there was only a tiny chance of this giving him more time, Dad wanted to try it. He also wanted the opportunity to help other people in the future. Unfortunately, this treatment made Dad very poorly and he turned bright yellow. At one of the hospital reviews with the oncologist there was a fruit stall just outside the hospital entrance. The fruit stall had a sign advertising the fruit it sold, the banner read 'Top Banana', with a picture of a lovely ripe banana on the front. Andrew had come with us and he asked Dad to stand by the sign so that he could take his photo. Dad had a great sense of humour and he stood there, bright yellow, with a big grin on his face next to the banana sign. It was a great photo and amongst other things, it illustrated the very close relationship between my Dad and Andrew.

Ultimately, it was obvious to me, and Dad also knew that he was going to die so we began to prepare. Dad found it comforting to talk to me about what would happen after the inevitable and I found that it also helped me to process the journey. Dad started by emptying the loft and shed. He did not want to leave us with things to sort out after he was gone. This behaviour is quite common when someone knows they are going to die, they tidy and prepare for death which gives them some control. He also told me where his hiding places were in the house for cash he had saved and proceeded to pull out rolls of money out of the radiators. There is nothing like preparing to die to make you and everyone around you aware of your own mortality. Talking to Dad about dying helped Dad and it certainly helped me which made the bereavement process easier. I don't think Mum took it on board though and I wasn't sure whether she was in denial. Dad was incredibly brave, he remained positive throughout and he never lost his sense of humour. We spent a lot of quality time together and I made him a promise that I would nurse him at home until his last breath.

Our family has always loved animals and we have always had pets but my love of equines is like an obsession. I have always been horse mad from the moment I could walk. During the time of Dad's diagnosis we had two horses - Aine a 16.2hh matriarch mare and Basil, my 17hh piebald beauty - both of them were competition Irish Sports Horses. We had owned Basil since he was 2 years old and I was the first person ever to ride him and we got Aine when she was 5 years old. Allister also had three donkeys, Lewella, Bryn and Amy. The equines lived as a herd outside in a large field with an open stable at my brother's house. Quality time for me and Dad meant caring for the horses and donkeys together and spending time outside. We both loved being outside and being with nature, passing time with the horses was therapeutic for us. We could chat about his illness in a way that was less intense and it felt more relaxed in this environment. Horses live in the moment, they don't think about yesterday or worry about tomorrow. We decided to live for the moment just like our horses during that time. That quality time together was incredibly special. I got to know the real man my father was, and to my surprise I found out that apparently he loved poetry. This was something that I never knew about him. One day we were walking around the field poo picking, the horses were wandering in amongst us and suddenly he would recite a poem. He would recite verses from lots of poems that were his favourites. He recited 'Leisure' by William Henry Davies to me and the words and the sentiment were profound. Davies describes modern life and how we are all rushing around and we no longer stop to appreciate the beauty of nature surrounding us. We all rush around and our focus is often on gaining material things and because of this we can become alienated from what is important. When Dad got his cancer diagnosis this poem summed up what is important in life and it is not the materialistic things that we often strive for. Dad found great comfort in his poetry. Mum less so.

'Bloody poetry, he is always reading bloody poetry.'

Not knowing that Dad loved to recite poetry made me reflect on how little we really know a member of our own family. Maybe that is because we have given them a job title, rather than seeing them as an individual. Dad was an incredible role model during this time, he managed to stay upbeat about life in the face of adversity and despite him being in the process of dying we would often joke and laugh together. I still treasure that quality time and having that time to make the most of the person whilst they are relatively well is the only benefit I can see of a cancer diagnosis. If anyone complained about the weather he would say, 'Every day is a good day.' As the cancer progressed, it was obvious that Dad was running out of treatment options as well as time, his organs were failing and he was slipping away from us slowly.

Mum and Dad met when they were very young, Mum was seventeen and Dad was eighteen when they started courting. Mum lived in a tiny village called Mount Pleasant in Mow Cop and Dad lived in another small village nearby called Dales Green. Although these two small Staffordshire villages were next to each other they didn't know each other because they attended different schools. When they met it was love at first sight and they started dating. Dad would tell me stories of how he would run across the fields to meet the bus that she was on, on her return from work. It was true love but unfortunately, they were soon to be separated because Dad had to join the army for his national service. National Service was a system of compulsory military service for a period of two years for young men in 1952, this conscription was necessary following World War 2, the Korean War and because of other military commitments abroad. Dad served his National Service mainly in Kent for two years. My parents were apart for most of this time except when Dad came home on leave. He would return on the train whenever he could, but Kent was 211 miles away from Mow Cop so it was infrequent. I remember Mum telling me tales of how she would be waiting to greet him at the train station with great excitement, when he returned home on leave. Dad was Mum's first and last boyfriend. They were very traditional in their views. Their parents were old fashioned and Mum had a very strict father. Dad told me that he had to build up the courage to ask Mum's father for his daughter's hand in marriage and how relieved he was when her father said, 'Yes.' They were granted permission to marry and they got married in a little church called St Luke's, just above Mount Pleasant in Mow Cop.

Mow Cop sits on a ridge at a height of 335 metres and splits two counties, Cheshire and Staffordshire. St Luke's church sits on the Cheshire side with beautiful views over the Cheshire plain. It is a beautiful small traditional grey stoned church which has a wild looking traditional grave yard. The church and its grounds seem sombre and yet majestic at the same time. The grave stones are very old and crooked, some of the graves are unkept and the people long forgotten whilst others are kept tidy and loved. The area has always reminded me of the film "Wuthering Heights" with its gritstone rocks, purple heather, moorland and wild weather. It is usually windy up there due to the height of the church in Mow Cop. My parents' wedding photographs looked so romantic with the backdrop of the old church and remoteness of the area. Mow Cop has a castle which can be seen for miles and dominates the landscape especially when viewed from the Cheshire side. The castle is a familiar site to anyone that lives on either side of the Staffordshire or Cheshire side of the ridge. Well, the castle is not really a castle, it is a folly, it was built as a summerhouse in 1754. It sits at 335 meters/1100 feet high in an exposed spot at the top of Mow Cop. It resembles part of a ruined castle and through time it has crumbled which has made it look slightly more ruined than its original build. It was constructed for Randle Wilbraham I, who lived at Rode Hall nearby on the Cheshire side. It was used for picnics by the family and visiting on days out. People continue to visit the castle for picnics and children scramble over the rocks. Allister and I loved climbing the rocks when we were growing up and visiting our Grandma. Mow Cop has a long history. It is said to have been a beacon point for the Romans which would have been used for communication and there is some evidence that the Romans lived in the area although this has not been confirmed. The land is rocky and made up of limestone and gritstone which was used for milling. This landscape gives the whole area an interesting and captivating feel.

In total, Mum and Dad were married for fifty nine years, like swans, together for life. They moved to Alsager, Stoke-on-Trent when they got married which is where they stayed and where my brother and then four years later myself, were born and grew up. My parents were the sort of couple that did everything together during their marriage, they enjoyed gardening, walking and dancing. They were loving parents and we were a very close family. As Dad prepared himself for death it was important to him that Mum was looked after following his passing away. His main concern was for Mum and never for himself. Just before Dad died he told me that he was worried about Mum. I told him not to worry and that I would make sure she was alright. He said, 'I know you will look after her but I think she is going funny just like her mother did.' Dad was probably the first one to diagnose Mum's dementia.

———◄►———

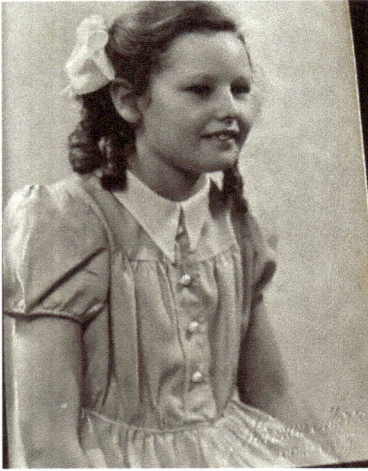

Sybil as a child approximate age 11 years old

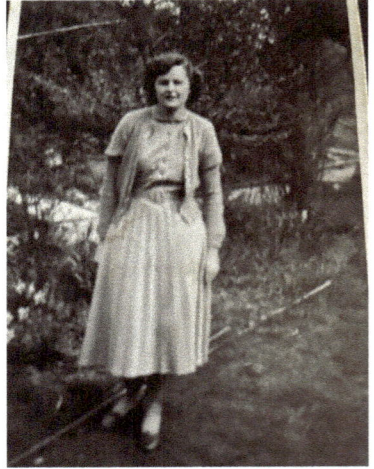

Sybil approximate age 17 years old

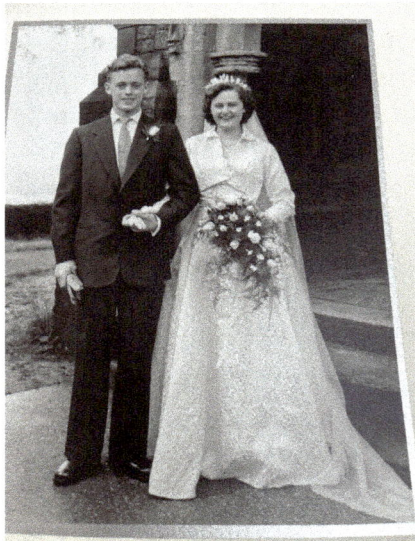

Alan and Sybil 20th July 1957

Chapter 2

Grandma Beech

My Grandmother on my mother's side, Amy Beech, known to Allister and me as Grandma Beech. Grandma Beech lived in a tiny house in West Street, Mount Pleasant, Mow Cop. It was a semi-detached house with two reasonably sized bedrooms which were accessed via a staircase going up in-between the two bedrooms. The stairs were very steep and enclosed with woodchip wall paper painted in magnolia. The bedrooms were decorated with wallpaper with a flower design. Grandma had a double bed with a mattress made of feathers. I used to stay over and sleep in this bed, I would sink down into the mattress which I found very comfortable. There wasn't a bathroom in the house which I found really strange. Downstairs consisted of a living room at the back of the house, a front parlour which was never used as it was saved for 'best'. The front parlour was decorated in large garish flowered wallpaper. There was a settee in there as well as a sideboard. 'Best' was never defined, although I had heard, that is where Grandad had been placed in his open coffin for a few days before his burial. That used to give me the heebie-jeebies, if I thought about the dead body for too long but luckily that was before I was born and at that point I had never seen a dead body. The front door was in the parlour but nobody ever used the front door unless someone had died and that's where they were taken out of the house as it was a special occasion. This all seemed very strange to me as a young child and it was enough to keep me out of the parlour. There was also a scullery downstairs where there was a sink for washing. The brick walls in the scullery were white washed. There was a toilet that could be accessed at the end of the scullery, this had been modernised apparently as the toilet used to be accessed from the outside and down the yard. The only room with any form of heating was the living room where there was an old fashioned grate and open fire. This room felt practical with woodchip wall paper, two armchairs, a small table with folding sides and two dining chairs. Next to and attached to the fire was a cast iron cooking range. Grandma would cook her food on this range as well as boil pans and her kettle. This is where Grandma and any visitors, unless they were posh visitors, which they never were, would sit. The room was my favourite as it was always warm and cosy, the fire was kept burning day and night. The coldest room was the scullery and there was no need for a fridge as the scullery and pantry were cold enough to keep food and milk fresh. When I went to the toilet, I would be as quick as possible so that I could get back into the warmth.

This house was my Grandmother's marital home and where my Uncle George was born and then a few years later in 1935, my mother was also born. Grandma Beech was widowed quite young and lived on her own for many years after Grandad's death. George Beech, my Grandad, had been a coal miner and his health had not been good for many years following an accident in the pit. He had experienced a crush injury that he had sustained when the pit roof had collapsed. He also had a poorly chest and suffered from pulmonary emphysema which was the cause of his death. The emphysema was attributed to his work in the pit but he also used to smoke Woodbine unfiltered cigarettes, so I was told. He was buried in St Luke's church and Grandma would often walk up the steep hill to the church to take flowers and to tend to his grave. She never remarried after his death and lived alone, although she came to visit us most weekends. Also, Uncle George, Aunty Dorothy and their son, my cousin Christopher lived in Mount Pleasant so she would see them regularly.

My first experience of dementia and particularly Alzheimer's dementia was with Grandma Beech. It was in 1978, when I was about twelve years old. Grandma was living alone in Mount Pleasant and all appeared to be well. However, strange behaviour started to happen when she was left alone. She had started to wander, this particularly happened in the evenings or at night, she would leave her house and wander around the village. Unbeknown to us, she was doing this a lot, even during the winter months. One winter evening, some school friends of mine were cruising around Mow Cop in a small group, there was very little to occupy teenagers in the village. Alsager was where a lot of the Mow Cop kids went to school and travelled to and from school every day on a school bus. This particular night, as they were walking past St Luke's church they spotted movement in the graveyard. They could see a pale figure floating along the path in and amongst the graves. They ran for their lives and only stopped when they got into the village centre. Curiosity then got the better of them and they decided to take another look, they walked up the steep hill and creeped back along aside the church wall. The ghostly figure was still there. They were about to run away again when one of my friends, Angela realised that this was not a ghost.

'It's Mrs Beech.'

They went over to speak to her and told her that she had given them the fright of their lives. Grandma was wandering around St Luke's church yard with her white hair, pale complexion in a floating white nightdress. Needless to say they thought they were seeing the spirit of a dead person.

Once they had realised that she was not a ghost, one of my school friends who lived in the same village recognised her and delivered her back to her house. My friend told me about this the next day at school and I told Mum. At the time I found the story about how Angela had seen and found Grandma in the graveyard quite funny. However, at the same time I remember that it felt embarrassing and I was ashamed. Mental illness carries such a stigma. I remember that there was great concern for Grandma's safety as she could have met anyone and not necessarily a friendly person. She was so vulnerable and she could have a fall and no one would know where she was. She could have got hypothermia and died as she was not dressed for the cold.

On another occasion, Dad had driven Mum and me up to Mow Cop to visit Grandma for the afternoon. We always went around the back of the house to the back door. As we entered we were presented with the sight of a buffet in the scullery. Grandma Beech had made sandwiches for Grandad ready for him to take to work down the pit. I found this to be bewildering as a child because my Grandad had died a year before I was born. I didn't know much about him apart from his reputation of being strict, being a coal miner and that he died of emphysema. Anyway, on the day that Grandma had made the sandwiches there was enough food to feed the whole mining workforce and not just Grandad. There was a long discussion as to why there were so many sandwiches, how many we could eat and what we were going to do with the surplus. Mum had to go around the neighbours offering the freshly made sandwiches. This was very confusing for me at the age of twelve years old as I had never met anyone with mental illness at that point. I did find the sandwich making incident mildly amusing but I tried to contain this amusement as I could see that it was upsetting for my Mum.

My Dad and I used to go to Grandma's to pick her up and bring her down to Wesley Avenue, Alsager where we lived at that time. We started to visit or to pick Grandma up more frequently following the sandwich and church incidents. One day we arrived at Grandma's house to find her locked inside the house. Through the closed window she told us that Grandad had locked her in and gone to work down the pit. She looked terribly distressed and all red in the face. Grandma Beech was cursing her husband for being mean and locking her in, the air was blue. Obviously, swearing was a family trait and inherited from Grandma Beech. Dad peered through the door lock hole and he could see that the key was on the inside but Grandma had turned the key and locked it from the inside and so preventing us entry. Dad looked puzzled and tried to push the key out of the back of the lock onto the floor to no avail. Dad looked like he was playing charades with lots of gesturing, mouthing instructions and acting out movements. I remember being very cold as we stood there with the wind blowing a gale. Mow Cop always seemed to be windy, wet and cold. It took about another hour to get Grandma to go to the back door and to turn the key, then she claimed that Grandad was playing tricks on her. We took Grandma to Alsager for the day. The situation was becoming a strain with constant visits to Mow Cop and these events were a great worry for Mum. There was no way of knowing whether Grandma was safe and she didn't have a telephone so we couldn't phone her either. Telephones were not a thing in those days because there were very few telephone lines and also Grandma couldn't afford one, let alone know how to use one.

The final straw came when Grandma fell down the steep stairs. Luckily, she didn't break any bones, she was just badly bruised and shaken up. Following the fall, it was decided that something had to be done. Grandma Beech was terrified of having to go into a nursing home which she called 'the workhouse' and she did not want to leave her own home. A workhouse was an institution that was intended to provide work and shelter for poverty stricken people who had no means to support themselves. People often became prisoners of the systems where people who were the most vulnerable in society were kept. They were worked hard for very little food or comforts. There was a real fear of workhouses and a great stigma was attached to them as well. The last Victorian workhouses closed following the birth of the NHS in 1948 and the Housing Act of 1949. Grandma was born on 29th December 1899, so she would know all about the workhouses. Grandma viewed nursing homes as workhouses and so did my Mum for that matter. So a nursing home was out of the question, however, it was clear that Grandma could not live alone any longer. Our house in Wesley Avenue, Alsager, was larger than Grandma's house but it was still a small three bedroomed semi-detached house. All three bedrooms were occupied by my parents, Allister and me. The access to upstairs also had a very steep staircase similar to Grandma's which wasn't really suitable for an elderly person. However, my parents decided that Grandma could no longer live alone and would come to live with us. I moved into Allister's bedroom, it was decided that my brother could sleep downstairs and Grandma would sleep in my small box room. We were the sort of family that came up with solutions.

So, Grandma came to live with us and her house in Mount Pleasant was sold. Grandma coming to live with us didn't quite work out as we expected. To understand why the transition was tricky, you have to look at the difference in the two houses. Grandma's house in Mount Pleasant never had a proper bathroom, she only had a sink and a toilet. There was no bath or shower in her home. A proper wash at Grandma's meant stripping off completely and washing at the sink in the downstairs bathroom. Having a bath consisted of a metal tub in front of the coal fire which was filled with water that was heated on the open fireplace. The house did have running water and a flush toilet but no other 'mod cons'. Once the water for a bath was heated up on the coal fire stove and it was tipped into the small oval tin bath, you could then have a bath but only if you were small enough to fit in. I used to love having a bath at Grandma's when I was small, sitting in the bath tub in front of the fire. It was wonderful, cosy and felt like a real adventure but I had grown too big to fit in by the age of twelve. When I was younger and smaller, I could sit for hours watching the flames dancing and imagining what I could see as the flames created shapes. The flames danced and told their own story as the shapes fuelled my young imagination. I have very special memories of my time staying with Grandma Beech prior to her becoming poorly and confused. We would toast bread on the open fire or we would cook jacket potatoes in the embers. We would have lots of fun whilst she would try to teach me some of the Mow Cop/Stoke dialect. Her favourite saying was;

'Koss Kikka bow, genst a wow an yeddit tillit bost.'

She would say it and I would repeat it, both of us laughing at how funny it sounded. This is an old common saying for anyone who has lived in Mow Cop or in the Stoke area and it is passed down through the generations. I don't know why it is said or where it originally came from but you often hear it in the area. It means;

'Can you kick a ball against a wall and head it until it bursts?'

Grandma never had a television, she lived a very simple and humble life. As a child I had noticed that Grandma used to talk to herself a lot and I thought that this was because she had lived alone for a long time. So living in Alsager was very different from what she was used to and all of the modern appliances were quite alien to her. I think these differences are what caused a few problems when she came to live with us.

I moved into my new bedroom and Mum and Dad bought a sofa bed for Allister so that he could sleep downstairs. Allister would have been 16 years old at this time and he had just started an apprenticeship. Whilst Allister was sleeping downstairs before going to work, Grandma would come downstairs at about 5am and proceed to strip off ready for a strip wash in the sink. As you can imagine this was to his horror, an older lady stripping off in front of him and especially as this was his Grandma. Something had to be done and fast. My Dad decided that a gate at the top of the stairs similar to that of a baby gate but homemade was the best solution. It would also prevent Grandma from falling down the stairs especially if she was going to descend the steep stairs in the dark in the middle of the night. Dad was a great carpenter and could make anything. He made a wooden gate which was erected and fastened at the top of the stairs which meant that Allister could sleep soundly without the early morning stripper appearing. Grandma however, was not too keen on the gate and used to give it a good rattle which would disturb everyone else in the house. Mum used to have to keep getting up to escort Grandma back to bed with lots of 'Shush, you will wake everyone,' and Grandma would reply in a loud voice 'I Wunna! Shush.' Grandma spoke a lot in the Staffordshire, Mow Cop dialect and more so when she was cross. Wunna means I will not. She could be very feisty which was put down as being part of the dementia .

Somewhere around this time in 1978, Grandma was diagnosed with Alzheimer's dementia. I can't remember how this was diagnosed and this was before fancy scans were available or even invented. As young people do, I would observe her behaviour closely with quizzical interest. I worked out that a person living with dementia commonly does things that seem strange to others, however, to fully understand what and why they are doing strange things, you need to look back into that person's past. It made sense to Grandma Beech to strip wash at our kitchen sink because she had never had a bath or shower at her house. Lots of strange behaviour seemed to make sense once I applied this theory. Grandma used to vacuum the carpet with the vacuum in one hand and the plug in the other or she would use a brush and pan to clean the carpets. I realised that this was because Grandma had previously only ever owned a mechanical push along Ewbank carpet cleaner, she had never owned a vacuum cleaner. A vacuum cleaner was seen as a luxury and a modern appliance by Grandma. So every morning whilst I was getting ready for school, Grandma used to push the unplugged vacuum cleaner around me whilst telling me that the vacuum cleaner was not picking up any bits off the carpet. She informed me that these modern day appliances were not as good as the old fashioned Ewbank's and she didn't know why my mother was wasting her money buying one. I used to try to explain about plugging in the vacuum cleaner but every day was like ground hog day and the new information was never retained. This particular activity of hoovering used to frustrate and aggravate me, I could feel the irritation creeping through my body as she pushed the vacuum around and I just couldn't wait to get out of the house and go to school.

My Mum worked part-time as a Caretaker in a local primary school at this time. We were a typical working class family who never had a lot of money but as children we never wanted for anything either. My parents were both hard working. Dad worked in a factory which didn't pay that well, so Mum had to work part time to earn some extra money. Mum could not afford to give up work, therefore Mum had to leave Grandma alone in our house for two hours in the morning and for two hours in the afternoon until I came home from school. It wasn't all bad though, Mum realised that Grandma could be an asset with the household chores and was much calmer when she was kept busy. Grandma was great at doing jobs such as cleaning the brasses. So the brasses would be put on top of the table on some old newspaper along with the Brasso metal cleaning polish and some old dusters. Grandma would set to with rubbing Brasso on with a duster and then polishing away. We had the cleanest brasses in Alsager. The only problem with this is that she was a very quick and efficient worker which meant that the cleaning brasses job did not last two hours. Grandma wanted to help around the house and do more chores. She thought she was being helpful and therefore she would look for other ways in which she could help Mum.

Mum came home from work one day to find that Grandma had been cleaning and peeling some potatoes for dinner. Our family loved potatoes and we would eat them most evenings, sometimes we would have mash, and sometimes we would eat roast potatoes, or chips for a change. There was one problem though. Grandma was also efficient at cleaning and peeling potatoes, she had peeled every potato in the bag. Dad used to buy the potatoes from the local farm to save money and the bag weighed 25kg. There were potatoes overflowing in every bowl, bucket, kitchen vessel and saucepan that Mum owned. Mum was presented with enough potatoes to feed the whole street. Grandma's hands were cold, white and wrinkled from the hours she had spent with her hands in cold water peeling the spuds. She looked very proud of her effort though and could not understand Mum's reaction. Mum burst into tears and Grandma just said,

'What are you blarting for, it's only potatoes?'

"Blarting" is an old fashioned word used in Staffordshire meaning crying. Mum took a few deep breaths and pulled herself together. I was then sent around to all of the neighbours' houses offering them peeled potatoes. The potatoes did not go to waste and the neighbours loved having peeled potatoes presented to them after a busy day at work but for Mum and Dad this was an expensive day. This was a very costly enterprise which could not be repeated.

On another occasion, Mum came home to find her saucepans burning on the open fireplace. The smell of the burning enamel was sickly. In Grandma's mind she had been helping again and had peeled the vegetables in preparation for dinner but she had put the pans of vegetables onto our coal fire. Our coal fire was not designed for cooking on. Again this made sense to Grandma, if you looked back into the past; she did not have a cooker, she had an oven and hob which was part of the fireplace, a bit like a Rayburn oven but actually part of the fireside. In Mount Pleasant, she had done all of her cooking on an open stove which was part of her hearth. On this occasion not only was the food ruined, all of the saucepans were burnt but more seriously we realised that the house could have been set on fire. Grandma Beech could not comprehend what the fuss was about. The final kitchen drama came when Grandma had tried to be helpful again in getting food ready, she had remembered the fuss about cooking on the fire so she had decided to use the kitchen gas hob. She put the vegetables into pans and place them on the gas hob, however, she never lit the gas ring. The house was gradually filling with gas. Luckily Mum came home just in time to a smell of gas and she quickly switched off the gas cooker and opened the doors, thankfully there was no explosion. Again, something had to be done or there could be very serious consequences. It was decided that a cooker guard was required, this was needed to stop Grandma from turning on the gas and also needed to be made of something flame retardant. Dad fashioned the guard in metal in his workshop in the garage which was then placed over the gas knobs. This was ingenious and prevented the accidental switching on of gas. There was still a lot of nervousness about the hour that Grandma was left alone when Mum left for work and prior to me returning from school, so another gate was made by Dad and erected to prevent kitchen entry. Grandma was not happy about the extra security and complained, 'You are treating me like a kid.' Gradually our house was beginning to resemble a prison. We could live with this though and we soon got used to all of the gates and guards.

Life was fairly tough for my parents. There was no spare money for any help or care and there was no social or financial support so the burden fell to my parents and myself. I became a part time unpaid carer for my Grandma at the age of twelve years old but I enjoyed being with Grandma and I liked helping Mum, so I didn't mind. I also found Grandma Beech's antics amusing, there was never a dull moment once Grandma had come to stay. My parents did not get the opportunity to go out very often but they loved dancing so they asked me if I would mind staying in with Grandma. They started to go out dancing once a week in the evening and I would care for Grandma. Mum and Dad did sequence dancing which is a type of ballroom dancing. I loved looking after Grandma but it could be very challenging in the evening. The difficulty came because she would insist she was babysitting me. 'Come on it's past your bedtime.'

She would be trying to send me to bed but I really needed her to go to bed so that I could have some peace and watch television. Caring for or being with someone with dementia is extremely tiring and can lead to what may be seen as dishonourable behaviour by the carer. I used to try to persuade her to go upstairs to bed but she would refuse. We would end up arguing about who was supposed to be going to bed. So, I developed a cunning plan to get Grandma upstairs which on reflection seems quite cruel but it was a coping mechanism for me in this situation and it worked a treat. There was no help or guidance provided on how to manage or care for a relative with dementia who was living with you. There were no support groups as there is now, you just had to work it out as you went along. My plan worked every time. I would throw Grandma's slippers upstairs, then run upstairs and hide behind my bed. She would follow me upstairs to retrieve her slippers, cursing me along the way. I would hide until she went past me on the landing, I would then quickly sneak downstairs, closing and locking the upstairs gate behind me. Once Grandma was upstairs she would rattle the gate, telling me,

'What a naughty girl you are,' or she would say, 'You are peevish,' and then she would tell me how she would tell my mother what I had done when she got home. However, once she was upstairs she would settle and go to bed.

Grandma was a very active lady and she would frequently wander at night, she would shake and rattle the gate. We were all sleep deprived for many years. Grandma was also very agile even in her old age and she could walk for miles without getting tired. Sometimes she would become very disturbed and troubled due to the dementia. Being restricted from leaving the house for safety reasons especially when she was left alone made her agitation worse. Sometimes she would become very distressed which is part and parcel of dementia. Grandma would insist that she was going to go home to Mount Pleasant so that she was there for when Grandad came home from work. We tried reasoning with her but she just insisted on leaving.

'I just wanna go wom,'

Grandma spoke with her broad Mow Cop accent. Wom means home and is a Stoke dialect. She would say that Grandad would be very angry if he came home to nothing for his supper. The trouble with this was she no longer had a home to go home to. Trying to tell someone with dementia that they no longer live in the house that they believe is theirs or trying to tell them that their husband died is a waste of time. Their belief in what they are thinking is so strong and real to them, that to them, it is real! Therefore, It is very difficult to know what to say to the person with dementia as telling them the truth can be very traumatic and cause extreme stress. A good example to explain this is for you to imagine that you have children who have to be picked up from school at 3pm. Then someone tells you that you cannot leave. You are then prevented from leaving by this person and then they tell you that you don't have any children or that your children have grown up and no longer go to school. What would you do? How would you behave? Would you become aggressive in an attempt to pick up your children? It is very likely that you would become very distressed but you may also become violent because you truly believe that you need to go to pick up the children. Well, Grandma insisted she was going home to see and feed Grandad. Initially, we tried to distract her to prevent her from wanting to leave but this did not work and caused high levels of anxiety and distress. So we decided to let her leave to go home. She would get her coat and shoes on and leave through the back door, thanking us for having her and saying that she would see us again soon. At first, we would follow her and check she was going in the right direction. The distance from Alsager to Mount Pleasant is approximately six miles, this included busy main roads as well as tiny country lanes and there is a very steep two mile hill at the end of the walk. Grandma would set off at a good pace and surprisingly she seemed to know where she was going. She followed the same route every time. So we would let her walk, my parents would telephone a family friend who lived at a farm approximately three miles away. When Grandma went past the farm we would get a phone call to say she had passed the farm and then Dad would set off in the car to pick her up. He would know her exact route, so he would drive that way and when he caught up with her he would wind his car window down and ask her if she wanted a lift. She would reply,

'Oh, hello Alan, I'm so glad to see you, the buses are on strike and I'm so tired.'

She would then get into the car and be content. She had managed to walk approximately five miles. Now that she had expelled her built up energy she would be calm and Dad would turn the car around and bring her back home to Alsager. This was a high risk strategy from a safety point of view but one that worked every time and was much better than the battle and chaos of trying to prevent her from leaving.

Unfortunately, Grandma put her ability to walk into action when Mum and Dad were offered one week's respite care for Grandma in hospital. Grandma was admitted into the elderly care unit at Leighton hospital in Crewe but she had other ideas than to stay there. Grandma could read the signs 'Way Out' and she kept escaping from the hospital ward. Of course they couldn't cope with this as they were short staffed and so they drugged her to prevent her from wandering. Following our family holiday, my parents went to pick up Grandma from the hospital to find her drugged and docile. When Mum saw her mother in a catatonic state she was extremely upset as she never believed in drugging Grandma. Needless to say that was the end of family holidays.

On the odd occasion my parents would take Grandma and myself out with them to the local sequence dance. Dad would go to the bar to get the drinks in, I would have a Coca Cola and Grandma would have a single whiskey. I had never really seen Grandma with a drink of alcohol before so it was quite a shock when she knocked it back in one go and asked for another and then another. Oh boy, could Grandma drink whiskey. This was too expensive for my parents so from then on when they took Grandma out, they used to sneak in a hip flask of whiskey in Mum's handbag to top Grandma up. At home and on evenings where Grandma was agitated she used to insist on going to the pub. This was a revelation to me as I had never known Grandma to go to a pub. However, apparently in her youthful years she used to enjoy a tipple of whiskey in the Robin Hood pub at Rookery. Rookery is another small village close to Mow Cop. Anyway, she used to insist on leaving the house to go to the pub. Again, at first Mum and Dad were reluctant to let her go as they thought this would mean another car trip to Mow Cop and it was not safe for Grandma to walk in the dark especially down country lanes. I would be involved with these struggles and I would try to help to distract Grandma but it was no use so we had to let her go. Again, we made sure she was dressed for the weather and off she would go. To our surprise though she left via the back door and would walk around to the front of the house, knock on the front door. Mum would answer the front door, greet Grandma as if we hadn't seen her in a while, hang her coat up and she would come in to the front room. Mum would hand Grandma a glass of whiskey and she would sit contently drinking her tipple. The front room was one long room which was also part of the dining area, Dad had knocked the middle wall down to make the house look more spacious. After a couple of hours and several whiskeys, Grandma would announce that she had to leave to go home, she would go into the hall, put her coat on, leave via the front door and return via the back door. I found this highly amusing and entertaining. On her return I would ask her how the Robin Hood was and had she enjoyed herself? She would reply saying that she had. We learnt to accept the Alzheimer's dementia and how to work around it, sometimes there was laughter and sometimes there were tears but one thing was consistent and that was love and a shared caring responsibility in our family.

Grandma Beech lived with us for approximately four years. Gradually she became more dependent on Mum in every activity of daily living. She eventually became less mobile, more confused, doubly incontinent and frail. Mum made sure she was always clean and immaculately dressed. With frailty comes the risk of infection. Grandma eventually succumbed to a nasty chest infection which then turned into pneumonia. Grandma died peacefully in our home in my old bed in the single box room. What really surprised me is that the day before she died she became completely lucid with no sign of the dementia. Apparently, this is a phenomenon called terminal lucidity which is very common. During this period of lucidity, Grandma thanked Mum for looking after her so well and said that she could not have done anymore. Uncle George was summoned to her bed side for one last visit where she informed him that he definitely could have done more to help Mum. I was there when Grandma died and although it was unpleasant to witness at such a young age I am grateful that my parents never shielded me from it. Grandma Beech was the first dead person that I had seen. I went into the room where she lay and touched her. Her arm was cold, it had a waxy feel to it and to me it no longer felt human. I have never forgotten this experience and that feeling of when a person dies they really have left their bodies and the body is just an empty shell. When Grandma Beech was still living, she was always warm to touch and her body was full of life, this was no different when Alzheimer's invaded her brain. Caring for Grandma Beech and having this deep insight into dementia turned out to be invaluable later on during my nursing career and also whilst caring for Mum when she also got diagnosed with Alzheimer's dementia.

Chapter 3

Nursing

From the early age of four years old, I had known what I wanted to do when I was older. I was going to be a nurse, there was no doubt about it. This early interest started when my Dad broke his leg badly in a terrible motorbike accident. He spent months in hospital waiting for his bones to heal and to knit back together. The accident had occurred when Dad was on his way to collect Grandma Beach from Mount Pleasant on his motorbike and sidecar. We didn't have a car at that time so we used to all sit in the sidecar whilst Dad rode his motorbike. We couldn't afford a car. I usually went with him to collect Grandma but on this particular day I didn't go with him. On his way to Mount Pleasant there is a very narrow and bendy road called The Hollows. A car was coming down this small lane at speed and ploughed straight into the side of Dad's motorbike, crushing him against a stone wall. He sustained a broken femur, tibia, fibula as well as crushing his patella. People rushed out of the houses nearby to help him. They laid him flat on the cold tarmac where he lay waiting for the ambulance. Then they thought he would be more comfortable sitting in a chair so they picked him up and placed him on a dining chair. Well as you can imagine, he screamed to be put back onto the floor. They placed him back on the cold floor where he proceeded to go into shock. The ambulance arrived and rushed him to the North Staffs A&E department where he was assessed and rushed to theatre for emergency surgery because he was losing a lot of blood.

He had lost so much blood that he nearly died. At first they thought he would lose his leg but the surgeon managed to save it. Allister & I were at home waiting for Mum or Dad to come home. The strangest thing happened which I have always remembered. Allister burst into tears moments before a police car appeared in our Avenue. I was four years old and Allister was eight years old, we were home alone. In those days there wasn't an age limit of being allowed to be left without an adult in attendance. Presumably he was looking after me whilst we were waiting for Mum to come home from work. I was asking him what was wrong and why he was crying when a policeman knocked at the front door. We were asked to go to our next door neighbour for the next few hours because Dad had been in an accident and Mum had been taken to see him. Allister has never been able to explain how he knew something was wrong and it was long time before we even had a telephone. Mum was eventually driven home in a police car.

Mum didn't and couldn't drive and she went through her whole life without ever learning to drive. Mum would have to use the public transport to visit Dad with me aged four and Allister aged eight in tow. We used to catch the bus twice a week to travel from Alsager, up to Hanley and then we would catch another bus to Newcastle. This was a major effort for Mum with two small children but she always made the effort to visit. I don't remember the long journey to get to the North Staffs Royal Infirmary in Newcastle, Stoke-on-Trent but I do remember the ward. I remember the smell of Dettol disinfectant and the strange clinical odour. I also remember seeing my Dad's leg which was stuck in the air with ropes and a pulley, providing traction to pull his leg straight, with weights hanging from the bottom of the bed. He had metal pins sticking out of his leg which were attached to metal bars and there were patches of brown iodine around the holes where the pins went into his skin. I instantly fell in love with the nurses' smart pristine uniforms, the starched hats and the disinfectant smells on the ward. I didn't feel scared by the pins sticking through Dad's leg or the other sights that I saw on the ward. I felt comfortable there, it was where I wanted to be and I knew that this is what I wanted to do, right from that moment. I remember telling Mum and Dad that I wanted to be a nurse, so Dad told me that I had better get my name put on the waiting list straight away. So I confidently went up to the nurses' station and asked the nurse in charge if she could put my name on the waiting list to become a nurse. The nurse took my name and date of birth and added me to the said list. It was many years later at high school that I realised that Dad had played a trick on me by telling me that there was a waiting list. However, by then I was still determined to become a nurse. I took and passed the exams I needed and applied to be a student nurse.

Eventually in 1984, when I was eighteen years old I left home to start my nurse training at the North Staffs Royal Infirmary. Both of my parents had always encouraged my desire to become a nurse. Dad said that I would never be out of work as a nurse as they would never be able to replace that job with robots. Mum had also encouraged me to become a nurse but when I look back I believe she had a hidden agenda which was so that I could care for her in her old age. Mum used to tell me that it was an expectation for a daughter to care for her parents and she made it very clear that she never wanted to go into a nursing home. I loved my nurse training, the checked uniform and starched hats. The other student nurses in my set became good friends with our shared experiences. We worked on different wards, in different specialities and every eight weeks my nursing set (84/5S) returned to the classroom for two weeks of theory before returning to different nursing specialities. Our nurse training was strict but we gained a good grounding for the future in our nursing careers.

A year after I had left home to go to live in the nursing home, Mum and Dad moved house. They moved out of our humble little house in Wesley Avenue which is where I was born and had grown up to a more 'modern' house in Eaton Road, Alsager. This house was a bigger three bedroomed semi-detached house with a beautiful garden and lots of space. My parents loved this house and made lots of good friends with the neighbours immediately. Mum and Dad were always willing to help other people and they seemed to fit in really well into their new neighbourhood. They both loved the big garden at the back of the house where they had a small vegetable plot as well as a Greenhouse. Dad had a large shed built in the garden so that he could continue with his wood crafting and DIY. They were both very house proud and used to do all of the decorating together. As soon as they had finished decorating the house, they would start all over again. The house was kept clean and tidy. When you went to visit there was always the smell of freshly baked bread, scones or cakes coming from the kitchen. The garden was immaculate, the lawns were mowed with stripey lines and the flower beds were a show of different colours. The flowers included marigolds, pansies, geraniums and peonies. The bees loved this garden with all the flowers for pollination. They would buzz about, darting from one type of flower and onto the next. The garden was always full of wildlife due to the bird feeders strategically placed in view of the house. There were Blue Tits and chaffinches galore. There was also the urban squirrel population that do so well, from the British gardens, and bird feeders. Our family dog, Mickey and the cat, Jaz, lay on the freshly mowed lawn and the whole picture was a vision of harmony and happiness.

My Dad's father, Grandad Boote was 82 years old when he came to live with Mum and Dad following a fall down the stairs in 1988. He had come home from the pub to his small house in Dales Green, slightly drunk. He had taken himself off to bed but on his way he had somehow fallen down the stairs. He was taken to the North Staffs A&E department where I was working as a staff nurse. Following an X-ray he was told he had broken his neck and needed to be admitted to the Orthopaedic ward. Whilst he was in hospital I used to visit him at lunchtimes on the ward to feed him as he was lying flat. After a few months of spinal traction on a Spiker bed and a few weeks recuperating he was allowed to leave to come and live with Mum and Dad. Due to the months of reduced mobility, he was rigid with arthritis, totally immobile and quite frail but mentally alert. Mum and Dad's house was not ideal for an old person with mobility problems but again, they made it work. The dining room was turned into a downstairs bedroom. A hospital bed and hoist were loaned to them so that they could move Grandad in and out of bed. Grandad lived with my parents for about five years. He loved Mum's cooking and would often praise her culinary skills. He didn't have much of a quality of life due to his immobility but up until that point of his life he had enjoyed an active life as well as a drink of beer. He had worked all of his life and when he was eighty years old he was still helping out on a local farm in Dales Green where he lived. So when he came to live with my parents he was content to just be still, he enjoyed looking out through the patio doors into the garden and watching the birds. The family dog and cat would keep him company. Grandad did eventually have to move to a peripheral hospital for the last six months of his life though because he became so immobile he could no longer be transferred to a chair. Dad tried to manage with the hoist for a while but eventually Dad had to admit defeat. Grandad died peacefully in one of the old peripheral hospitals. There were many of these old peripheral hospitals in Stoke-on-Trent and although they were dated, they provided an invaluable service to the NHS and they also helped to free up hospital beds.

There was never any regret for my parents caring for Grandma Beech and Grandad Boote. They were glad to have taken on the responsibility. There has been an unwritten rule in our family that you cared for your relatives when they got old. I always felt that this responsibility would come my way and it would be expected of me to care for my parents when the time came, especially with me being a nurse. I didn't think that this would ever be Allister's role. So when Dad was diagnosed with cancer, it was only natural that I became his carer and nurse. My nursing background was invaluable during this time. The last few weeks of Dad's life were pretty traumatic. His legs had become so swollen due to organ failure that he could hardly lift his legs off the ground when walking and all of his bodily fluids were pooling in the lower half of his body. I had to go to Marks & Spencer's to pick up some enormous jogging bottoms and pants as he couldn't fit into any of his clothes. The cancer was infiltrating his vital organs but he kept on fighting. His only concern was for Mum being left alone after he died which he knew was approaching soon and he was powerless to stop.

One day, I got a phone call from one of his neighbours to say that Dad had collapsed in the kitchen and an ambulance was on its way. I rushed over to their house and got there just as the paramedics arrived. Dad had a huge gash in his head that needed stitches. Dad was taken to Leighton hospital in Crewe. I followed the ambulance in my car and met Dad there. I thought we would be there for hours so Mum stayed at home. However, Dad was triaged and seen by a doctor very quickly because of his head injury plus he looked extremely poorly, he was bright yellow by this time due to the cancer in his liver. I consulted with the doctor;

'Please could you stitch my Dad's head up so I can take him home?'

'He needs a CT scan because of his head injury.'

'Really, well what exactly are you going to do with him if he has a fracture of his skull? I don't mean to be funny but he is dying and I want to take him home!'

'We really need to do a CT scan.'

'How long is the wait for this as time is extremely precious to him?'

The doctor looked at me as if I had lost my mind. We waited for only a short time and Dad had his CT scan. I think they put him through as a priority. The hospital were great and I think they rushed him through because of how poorly he actually was. The CT scan showed no brain damage, it was normal, thank goodness. Dad's head was stitched up and then I wheeled him to my car to take him home. It took Dad and me ages to get him in the car, the weight of his legs which were full of fluid was so heavy he couldn't lift them and they had started to leak clear fluid out of the pores. I had to climb onto the back seat and pull him in, he then had to sort of lie on the back seat because of his gigantic legs. Mum was there waiting for him at the front door. A sandwich and a cup of tea were soon produced for both of us.

About a week later, Mum phoned me in the middle of the night to tell me that Dad had been to the toilet and the toilet was full of blood. She was distraught and didn't know what to do. I told her to keep Dad comfortable and not to flush the toilet as I needed to see what was passing through his body. Andrew and I rushed over in the car, going as fast as we could without breaking the law. When we got to him it was obvious to me that he was suffering from hypovolaemic shock. I went to have a look in the toilet which was full of blood and clots. Something had obviously ruptured inside his body. Going through my head was Dad's request to die at home but he really needed emergency fluids. Dad lay on the sofa, he was cold but clammy and shaking with a combination of fear and shock. I pulled up a stool and sat down next to him and held his hand. I asked him what he wanted to do, whether he wanted to stay at home which would probably mean the end of his life or whether he wanted to go to hospital for treatment and a drip. I made it clear that if he did go to hospital, he may not make it home this time. It was a terrible conversation to have but it needed to be said. He told me that he wanted to go to hospital and so I quickly called 999. Andrew sat holding Dad's hand whilst I stood in the hall to call and speak to the ambulance service. I have never seen my father scared in my whole life but that night, he was terrified. Soon there were sirens heading our way. When the paramedics arrived they wanted to take him straight away but Dad was worried that he needed the toilet again. Then he vomited some blood called coffee grounds. The paramedic and me looked at each other and the urgency was turned up a gear to get him into hospital. Mum travelled with Dad on this occasion as the paramedic thought that Dad may not make the journey. Andrew and I followed in the car. That was such an anxious journey. As soon as they got into the A&E department at Leighton hospital, Dad had lots of blood tests and they put an intravenous drip into him to stabilise him overnight. I could see that soon after giving Dad fluids he started to look more comfortable. The A&E doctor came and asked me if I was aware of how poorly he was and told me he probably only had a few days to live. I told the doctor that I was aware and of my Dad's wish to die at home. I asked the doctor to give me until the next day to sort a commode and a bed downstairs at my parents' home. I told them that when I was ready, I would phone them and could they please then provide an ambulance to bring him home. They told me that they could but only if I was sure I could manage because they could not arrange any nursing care as it was the weekend. I reassured the doctor that Andrew and I would nurse him. The next morning I called Douglas McMillan, Hospice at Home, who were amazing. Within a few hours a hospital bed and commode were delivered to the house. Hospice at Home was arranged which did not provide any nursing care but they did provide a person to be present in the day for support. This was great because they could sit and chat with Mum to take her mind off what was happening with Dad. The district nurse was available to provide regular Morphine pain relief. I called the hospital and as promised Dad was delivered home. In the front room was a hospital bed all made up and next to it was a commode. When the ambulance personnel wheeled Dad into the house on a stretcher and he looked into his front room he said,

'Somebody has been bloody busy!'

I did manage to fulfil my promise to Dad with the help of Andrew and we nursed him at home in his last few days. At night, I slept on the settee in the front room so that Dad was never left alone and this also allowed Mum to go to bed and to get some rest. Andrew stayed at my parents' and slept upstairs in case I needed him quickly. Dad still managed to keep his sense of humour and he even enjoyed an episode of Poldark on one of his last days on earth. On Dad's last evening, Andrew asked him how he was feeling, Dad smiled and replied 'Champion!' Allister had returned from holiday in Ibiza a day or so before. Myself, Mum and Allister were all present when Dad eventually took his last breath. Dad died at home on 25th October just as he had wished, in the comfort of his beloved home.

Once all the formalities were sorted with the funeral, Dad's death hit me like no other grief I had ever experienced. It was so painful both mentally & physically as well. I would experience a heavy type of sensation deep inside my chest which made it difficult to breathe. I had a deep burning sensation in my throat that was choking. The sadness that I felt was beyond profound. I believe that whilst he was still alive, I was his carer and nurse and therefore, I felt I had to be strong. This had kept me strong and practical. For example, it was I that was given the horrible task of discussing his non-resuscitation agreement. His own doctor should have done this but he had just made a complete mess of it by asking Dad outright over the telephone whether he wanted to be resuscitated or not. Dad had understood this, as the doctor wanting to stop all of his cancer treatment. Also following Dad's death, it was I that had to hold up Mum and sort out all of the practical elements of death and the burial. Therefore, once all of the practicalities were done and dusted, I was left with this huge emptiness. It was like standing on a cliff edge waiting to tip forward into the void. There seemed no time for my grief, I was needed by Mum more than ever but I was also the owner and joint director of an occupational health business. I had to be strong, keep a stiff upper lip and just get on with life. It was when I was in the car and on my own that I experienced the worst and extreme grief, it would just hit me and I would have to pull over. I would wail and scream in the car where no one could see or hear me. Then I would shake it off, put on the mask, smile and carry on. The one thing that I could hold on to though was that I had never let Dad down and I had kept my promise to him which was to nurse him at home. Dad was not alone when he died and this was important to me.

Once the funeral and all of the administration were sorted, it was time to focus on Mum. I remembered what Dad had said about her starting to get confused and 'going funny just like her mother had'. Looking back now to the time after Dad had died and Mum was living on her own, there were many early signs of Mum's dementia. I think Mum also knew that she had dementia but she had become very good at hiding any obvious signs. The Post-It notes had begun to multiply, they were found everywhere. Lots of them with the same reminders or telephone number written on them. The Post-It notes were a simple sign but there were others too. Mum had always been an avid lover of sport and followed Athletics and Cricket. In her younger years, she had loved to go to Old Trafford cricket ground to watch a match. She had gradually lost interest in following any sport and no longer really supported the cricket. She would still watch sport but she was more like a passive observer rather than an enthusiastic follower. She used to love watching 'A Question of Sport' and she could answer many of the questions but again she lost interest in the programme and when she did watch it, she no longer attempted to answer any questions.

The kitchen had always been Mum's domain and she loved to bake, she was well known for her Scones, Cup and Victoria Sponge cakes. She would always bring out cakes when she had visitors. Her Christmas cake was an old recipe which was rich and tasted amazing. Mum was a great host and loved to provide food for visiting guests. She prided herself on her good cooking skills and there was always something on offer. The oven was always on and the kitchen would smell amazing with freshly baked cakes and that would be enough to tempt you to eat even if you weren't really hungry. One day, Andrew and I visited and we were asked whether we wanted a piece of freshly baked lemon cake. 'Of course,' we said licking our lips in anticipation. I am particularly partial to cake, you could describe me as a cake addict. The cake was presented, it looked amazing, we both took a bite out of our slice at the same time. Andrew nearly spat his mouthful out and looked horrified when he started to chew. I began to chew my mouthful of cake and realised that there was something very wrong with it. It was very gritty and crunched when you chewed it.

'I can't eat this Mum,' I asked, 'what have you done to it?'

Mum stated in a stern voice,

'There is nothing wrong with it,'

and then smiling whilst biting into the cake and trying her hardest to keep a smile on her face she said;

'Mmm, it's lovely!'

I watched her trying to pretend that she was enjoying it whilst she was crunching through the piece of cake.

'It's not Ok, is it?' I laughed and asked, 'Are you telling me fibs?'

She continued to chew and swallow with a smile and then we all burst out laughing as she knew she had been caught out and that she was not enjoying it at all. What had happened to the cake to make it so inedible was that she had baked it with granulated sugar rather than castor sugar and although it looked amazing, it had a horrible gritty texture. Nothing ever went to waste though, so the cake was broken up and put on the bird table. The birds in the garden, the Blue Tits and Finches didn't seem to have a problem with it and it was soon gone. At the time I assumed that this was Mum improvising for not having the correct ingredients rather than her forgetting the recipe. It was becoming obvious that Mum was becoming less able in the kitchen. Mum would forget what she was doing or miss out ingredients, she found this extremely upsetting. Her well known scones became cardboard in texture and were very dry and rock hard. Sometimes she forgot to put baking powder into the recipes and her cakes wouldn't rise. This was horrible to witness as she became very tearful and distressed. However, she would try to cover up the fact that she could no longer remember how to bake. Over the next few months she slowly but surely stopped baking.

Mum had always been an incredibly talented knitter and she also loved to crochet. In the past you would be able to ask her to knit a jumper with a particular pattern on it and she would just create the pattern and knit the jumper. Mum had also taken on unusual knitting requests and orders. When I was twenty one, she had knitted an undercoat for my thoroughbred ex-race horse Oaksey, who felt the cold easily. She knit the coat in multicolours with all of her spare wool and it had a hood so that he could put his head through the hole, he loved that coat. I used to call it Oaksey's multicoloured dream coat. She also used to crochet hundreds of blankets for new born babies, dogs and cats and for anyone else who wanted one. However, after Dad had died she started to lose her stitches and eventually she also stopped crocheting or knitting. When I asked her about this, she told me that she had lost interest or that there were no babies to crochet blankets for anymore. This again was a coping strategy as she did not want to admit that she was struggling. She had also started to withdraw from conversation and could only really manage a functional dialogue. I noticed that she would not only repeat herself a lot but she also used to provide great detail as to what she was about to do as if it were to remind herself of what she needed to do. Sometimes this detail was quite personal and was about personal hygiene. I used to say,

'Too much information Mum, Andrew doesn't need to know that.'

⸺⸺•❦•⸺⸺

Chapter 4

Diagnosis

I found myself discreetly observing Mum's behaviour and kept thinking back to what Dad had said to me before he died. He told me that he was concerned that Mum was 'going the same way as her mother, "funny".' In 2017, I eventually decided to tackle the issue and told Mum that I thought she was becoming forgetful and that we needed to get her assessed. I didn't want to upset Mum or to make her worry but it was becoming clear that her cognitive functioning was reducing. I approached the subject sensitively and told her that there were a lot of medications now available that can help with memory. She must have known really because she never objected. So I booked an appointment with her doctor. The doctor asked Mum lots of questions about what time and day of the week it was, he asked her what was the month and the year. She got the day of the week correct but not the month or the year. I was aware that she was becoming forgetful but not knowing what month or year was both surprising and upsetting for me. He then asked her to draw a clock face and to put the big hand of the clock at twelve and the little hand at five to read 5 o'clock. She struggled to do this. He showed her pictures to identify general everyday items such as a fork which she managed quite well. He asked her to subtract 7 from a hundred and then keep going for as long as she could, she managed to get to 86. I had to laugh though when he asked her who the prime minister was and she did a typical cover up and said, 'It's that silly bugger, you know who I mean.' She managed some parts of the test really well such as her address and date of birth but she could not remember some things like what had happened to Dad. The doctor asked me questions about her ability in understanding and handling money. I told him that Mum could no longer go shopping on her own as she couldn't understand how much money to give at the till. Mum was referred to the Memory clinic to see a psychologist who specialises in memory and dementia. After a few weeks, we received a letter to attend the clinic. The Memory Clinic was at Bradwell Hospital in Stoke-on-Trent. I knew this hospital really well because it was my first post after qualifying as a Registered Nurse. The hospital had changed a lot but it brought back lots of happy memories for me. When the new Bradwell Hospital was first opened by Princess Diana in 1987, I was the first nurse that she met and talked to. She was so kind to the patients and they adored her, I still have the newspaper photograph of the occasion. Di and I were on the evening news together and in the local paper. The Memory Clinic was in a small corner of this hospital and ironically it seems like it was hidden away and forgotten, a bit like its patients. Dementia carries a stigma around wherever it goes and it is the poor relative of diagnostics. Anyway, we attended the appointment and Mum went through a series of cognitive tests similar to that ones that Mum's doctor had given her to do. She did slightly better and got a better score on this particular day. The specialist told us that she just had mild cognitive impairment due to ageing rather than dementia. The term 'mild cognitive impairment' is used when symptoms are not severe enough to be diagnosed as dementia. The specialist arranged for a further scan and a review in six months' time. We came away ecstatic that she had not received a diagnosis of dementia, it was a huge relief for Mum. However, inside, my intuition was telling me a different diagnosis. I was not totally convinced that this was not dementia as I had witnessed some strange behaviour and I wondered whether she was just having a good day.

Straight after the hospital appointment, I did arrange for Power of Attorney for finance and health whilst Mum still had the mental capacity and whilst Mum could still provide informed consent. I had been dealing with all of the finances and bills etc anyway ever since Dad had died. Mum had dealt with all of the household bills all of her married life but I had noticed that she was getting confused. She no longer seemed to understand money or how much anything cost including the bills. Mum and Dad were old fashioned and they had always paid the bills at the local Post Office. When I started taking care of the finances I changed the method of payment to direct debit which was so much easier.

Following Dad's death I had also started to take Mum shopping once or twice a week because she didn't drive and the weight of the shopping was too heavy to carry all the way back from the village centre. There was no way she could manage to do the shopping on foot. I liked shopping with Mum and I could also do mine at the same time so it made sense. Mum had been going to the local supermarket for years and she was well known by all of the staff there. Observing Mum at the checkout was an eye opener. Mum would put her shopping on the conveyor belt, the lady on the checkout would scan items whilst Mum packed her shopping into bags. All seemed well until the checkout lady on the till would tell Mum how much she owed for the shopping. I let Mum pay but I observed her closely. Mum handed over a £10 note and then she looked for clues on the shop assistant's face to see if that was enough, when the shop assistant repeated the amount she owed, she would hand over another £10 note, then another and she would keep going until the shop assistant smiled. The shop assistant was kind and never told Mum that she hadn't paid enough, she just repeated herself until she had sufficient money to pay. Mum was obviously covering up the fact that she had no idea of the value of money anymore. This made me realise how vulnerable she was to fraud and how lucky we were that the shop assistants knew Mum and were very honest. As a family we decided that Mum could no longer be trusted with paying any bills or with handling money and she would always need a chaperone for any shopping. At the same time, it was important that we tried to maintain Mum's independence whilst ensuring that she was safe.

My niece Hayley, got married in September 2017 and we attended the wedding at the church and reception. We all stayed at the hotel where the reception was. The hotel was lovely and modern but it was quite expensive. Andrew paid for two rooms, one for us and one for Mum. The next morning Mum gave Andrew the money for her room; £17.50. Andrew didn't know what to say so he thanked her and came to tell me that the room was £175.00 and he had been short changed. This was another confirmation that Mum had no idea about money anymore. Mum would move the decimal point either up or down. A person may benefit or lose out because of this. The Grandchildren could potentially receive 50 pence, £5, £50 or £500 as a birthday gift and she would have no idea of what she was giving them. The lack of understanding money was of great concern to us. I worried in case she needed to pay for anything in cash. Therefore, we had to ban Mum from going to the Post Office or shopping on her own. One day my son Cameron, took Mum to collect her pension from the local Post Office. He stood nearby to her, observing her closely to make sure she was doing everything correctly. She had her PIN number written down in her purse which again made her vulnerable. The Post Office counter lady knew Mum well and viewed Cameron with suspicion. She asked him to step back away from the counter twice. Cameron stayed put and more suspicious looks followed. She then asked Mum if she knew this young man, 'Oh yes, this is my bodyguard!' she told her proudly. 'This is my grandson, Cameron.'

The six months passed quite quickly and it was time for Mum's review with the psychiatrist. Mum attended a CT scan first and then we returned to the Memory Clinic for her review. This time I was armed with more evidence that things were not well with Mum's memory and it was my opinion that this was more than mild cognitive impairment. The specialist did some more dementia tests. It was very noticeable that the cognitive impairment had increased drastically. Mum was very defensive saying that there was nothing wrong with her but I think this was because she knew there was. She was asked to remember three simple words. The doctor told her that he would ask her to repeat these words later on. When she was asked to draw the clock, she refused and told the doctor that he was treating her like a child. She could not tell him what month or year it was. It was very hard for me to sit there quietly, it was natural for me to want to help her by prompting her or by answering for her when she was stuck on a question. Mum was shown some pictures of various animals and was asked what they were, she was very confident with dog and cat but she had no idea what a giraffe was. She kept saying,

'Well, I can see it but I can't think what it's called.'

I couldn't believe that a person could lose this type of information. It was like she had never seen one before and although I know that they are not common in everyday life, I couldn't get my head around the fact that she had no idea what it was. This animal had been wiped off Mum's hard drive. The doctor then asked her to recall the three words from earlier, there was no recall. The CT scan results confirmed that Mum did have changes in the brain which were visible. She was diagnosed with Alzheimer's dementia. Mum burst into tears, her brain had not lost the memory of her own mother and her battle with Alzheimer's disease. Mum knew what that looked like and she knew what was coming her way. She could see her future clearly at that moment. The diagnosis was extremely upsetting for both of us. I remember thinking I don't know what was worse - Dad's cancer diagnosis where there was at least some hope of a cure or this diagnosis when you are told there is no cure. Mum was prescribed several medications to try to slow down the brain's impairment and to sharpen up thinking. However, that was all that the psychiatrist could offer.

Dementia is not a disease itself. It's a collection of symptoms that result from damage to the brain caused by different diseases, such as Alzheimer's. Alzheimer's disease causes shrinkage called atrophy, the shrinkage is in the posterior part of the brain. In Alzheimer's disease, amyloid plaques are present which are abnormal deposits of protein which damage and destroy brain cells. There become neurofibrillary tangles in the brain cells. Brain cells require the normal structure and functioning of a protein called tau. In Alzheimer's, threads of tau protein twist into abnormal tangles inside brain cells, leading to the death of brain cells. Dementia symptoms can affect people differently, and everyone will experience symptoms in their own way. Common early symptoms of dementia may include: memory loss, difficulty concentrating, difficulty in carrying out familiar daily tasks, struggling to follow a conversation or finding the right word, asking questions repetitively, being confused about time and place and mood changes. Mum had all of these. Close family are usually the first to notice these symptoms so asking the family is an important part of the diagnostic process. Dementia is not a natural part of ageing. The most common cause of dementia is Alzheimer's disease. As dementia progresses, memory loss and difficulties with communication often become severe. In the later stages, the person is likely to neglect their own health, and require constant care and attention. The most common symptoms of advanced dementia include people not recognising close family and friends, not remembering where they live or where they are. Some people may eventually lose the ability to speak altogether and many people become less able to move about unaided. Therefore, some may eventually become unable to walk and require a wheelchair or be confined to bed. A significant number of people will develop what are known as behavioural and psychological symptoms of dementia. These may include increased agitation, depressive symptoms, anxiety, wandering, aggression, or sometimes hallucinations. Bladder incontinence is very common in the later stages of dementia, and some people will also experience bowel incontinence. Appetite and weight loss problems are both common in advanced dementia. Some people simply forget to eat or drink because they forget that they are supposed to or because they get distracted. In the later stages, many people have trouble eating or swallowing, and this can lead to choking, chest infections and other problems.

I started to look at the future and what Mum would need. Andrew and I decided that Mum would need to come and live with us eventually but we would try to maintain her independence for as long as possible. After all, I had made a promise to Dad to look after Mum and I intended to keep that promise. To begin with, Mum would remain in her home with regular visits from Allister and me and the grandchildren. Allister lived in Alsager and so he could call in to see Mum in the evening to make sure she was alright. I would go down several times a week and take Mum shopping on a Monday.

In the back of my mind, I also began to worry about my own future and whether dementia was going to be my destiny. I kept thinking of Grandma and then Mum. It is terrifying to consider that this is what is likely to happen to you and so I could understand Mum's distress. The doctor reassured me that Alzheimer's disease is not inherited and it is just a common disease. Because Alzheimer's disease is so common in people in their late seventies and eighties, having a parent or grandparent with Alzheimer's disease at this age does not change your risk compared to the rest of the population. However, there is conflicting information available about this and it is not entirely clear whether there could be a hereditary factor. The NHS website states that the genes you inherit from your parents can contribute to your risk of developing Alzheimer's disease, although the actual increase in risk is small. But in a few families, Alzheimer's disease is caused by the inheritance of a single gene and the risks of the condition being passed on are much higher. According to statistics published by the NHS, Alzheimer's affects around 1 in 14 people over 65 and 1 in 6 people over the age of 80. This equates to 850,000 people in the UK. Women are more likely than men to develop Alzheimer's, with women accounting for around 65% of cases of dementia in the UK. This has become a great concern for my brother and me considering that our mother and grandmother were both diagnosed with Alzheimer's disease and especially for me as a female. Despite this disease being so prevalent, it seems hidden away and carries an air of shame and humiliation. People seem to avoid talking dementia but maybe it's because it's too terrifying to contemplate as it could affect any of us. The statistics are powerful.

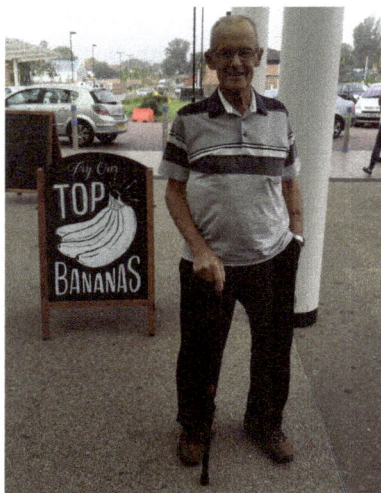

Dad with cancer bright yellow but he never lost his sense of humour

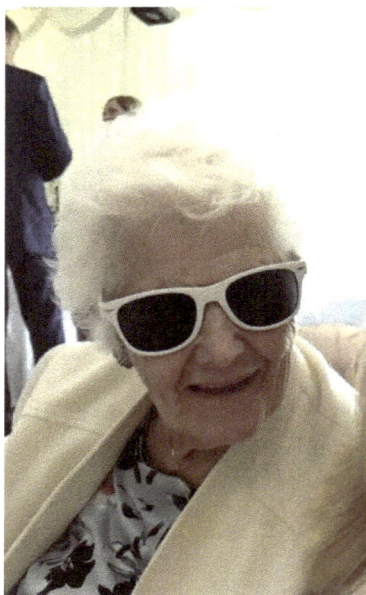

Mum at Hayley's and Craig's wedding 11th September 2017

Chapter 5

Lapwing Farm

Once I had realised that Mum needed more help and supervision because she was vulnerable, Andrew and I started to look for a house that would be suitable for when the time came when Mum would need to come and live with us. We both earned a reasonable wage and felt that we now could afford a house with some land so that we could keep our beloved horses at home instead of paying out lots of money for stabling and grazing each week. Having a house with its own land and stables would also mean that when Mum came to live with us, I wouldn't have to travel far for the horses, meaning that Mum would not be left alone for long. We decided that we needed a house that was reasonably close to Congleton, where we both worked. We worked together, we were owners and directors of an Occupational Health business. The house would need to have three bedrooms for us and our grown up boys, and a fourth bedroom for Mum that was going to be suitable for someone with disabilities. We wanted a minimum of two stables and enough land for the horses. A ménage would be great too, but not essential. A ménage is a riding arena which is well drained and has a suitable surface for riding. I had been keeping an eye on the property market for a couple of years at this point. Partly because it had always been my dream to own some land and to have our horses at home and partly because I was committed to having Mum come to live with us. Therefore, I was very aware of what houses were on the property market. About two years prior to Mum's diagnosis, I had seen a house for sale near to Leek in the Staffordshire Moorlands and I had fallen in love with it. However, the house was very expensive and more money than we could afford. The house would have been perfect though, it had a downstairs single room with a wet room suitable for a person with mobility problems, it had approximately fifteen acres with five stables and a menage. I remember telling Andrew that it was our dream house and then I had to forget about it as it was well above our budget.

I was doing my usual scanning of the property market in 2017. Whilst I was looking on Right Move, I was shocked to see that our dream house was on the market again. I jumped up and shouted for Andrew to come and look at the advert on the computer, especially as the house was about two hundred and a fifty thousand pounds less than it had been originally advertised. I could not believe that it was there and it matched every spec that we were looking for and so we enquired straight away. The estate agents told us that it was a repossession so it was owned by the bank. They warned us that it had been empty for approximately 10 months and that the electricity had been switched off and isolated, and the water had been drained off. We worked out that it was at the top end of our budget but we could afford it, so we arranged for a visit. The house sits between Rudyard and Longsdon on the outskirts of Leek in the Staffordshire Moorlands in a beautiful country lane. We drove up to the area which felt remote. However, Leek town centre is only 3 miles away which has all the amenities that we would require.

Leek is a lovely market town on the edge of the Peak District. The surrounding area is moorland and there is an impressive group of gritstone escarpments called The Roaches, Hen Cloud and The Ramshaw Rocks. The escarpment has a very distinctive shape with its edges and craggy rocks. The area is very popular with climbers as well as with walkers.

You can walk and clamber up on to the top of the escarpment through a well-used gap in the rocks, from there you can see for miles on a clear day. You can look out and see Tittesworth reservoir nearby and on a really clear day you can even see the mountains of Snowdonia in the far distance. The surrounding area is of marsh, bog and purple heather when it is in flower. The area has been designated as a Site of Special Scientific Interest (SSSI) and it is part of the South Pennine Moor Special Area for Conservation (SAC) due to its wildlife and habitat. The area is full of bird life which include Curlews, Red Grouse, Buzzards and in the cliffs there are Peregrine Falcons. So the area has plenty of interest from ornithologists and conservationists as well. Once you have reached the top of the escarpment, if you walk along the ridge you will reach Doxey Pool. This is a mysterious water body that looks black due to the peat and the ground that surrounds it feels hollow if you jump up and down. The pool can feel eery and at the same time magical, it is rumoured to be the abode of a mermaid who entices unsuspecting travellers to their watery end. A bit farther along is a trig point measuring trig the summit at 1,657 feet.

My parents used to take us up to The Roaches when we were children. We used to walk along to the Doxey Pool and as a child I remembered that I used to feel a sensation of fear and excitement. We would take a picnic and spend time climbing the different rock formations. Sometimes, we would continue along the rocky outcrop until we reached the road where we would continue straight on to Lud Church. Lud's Church is a steep chasm of rock located in the Dark Peak, hidden amongst the trees of the forest. It is an atmospheric, moss-covered chasm that hides plenty of secrets. The walls of the rock on either side stretch 59 ft up in the air, and are coated in sweet-smelling, vivid green moss. Lud's Church offers the perfect contrast to the rocky, open ridge of the Roaches. Lud's Church boasts a fascinating history, and over the centuries it has sheltered religious dissidents and political outlaws. In the 15th century, the Lollard followers of John Wycliffe used the chasm as a hiding place and a secret place of worship, hoping to avoid religious persecution. There are lots of stories about Lud's Church and it really catches people's imagination.

At the base of The Roaches is a house built into the rock which is called Rockhall Cottage. Nearby to this house is a secret spring well of water. When I was a child we used to spend hours in the garden of this house because my Mum and Dad became friendly with the man that lived there. My dad did some carpentry there and built the front door to the house. We used to play on the rocks in the garden and one of the rocks had footsteps cut into the rock so they were easy to climb. The house is now owned by the British Mountaineering Council (BMC) and has been renamed The Don Whillans Hut. Behind the house and all over the rocks you will see climbers enjoying The Roaches. The area is loved by many and has very special memories for Allister and me. My family used to visit the area every summer, we would walk and pick bilberries. There was lots of wildlife to see, if you were quiet you could see birds of prey, deer and wallabies. In the 1930s, five Australian Bennett's wallabies were released into the wild at The Roaches. This colony bred and their numbers grew, however, sadly the wallabies are said to have died out now and no one has reported seeing any for many years. I remember The Roaches with the sort of fondness that is built on foundations of childhood happy memories and of summer days of adventure. I have always felt drawn to this area because of the memories from my childhood. This was another sign that the house was right for us. Along the road you can see The Roaches and what a wonderful sight it is, it is particularly special when the light is right as it catches the heather and the rock. The rock seems to glow red, orange and yellow.

So we arranged to view the house. The house had stood empty for a while and appeared to be melancholy. It was a strange experience viewing the house as it felt isolated, cold and unloved. Every gate had been chained and padlocked. The electricity had been cut off and the water had been drained, leaving an extremely cold feel to the place. The small pond outside had been encircled with blue stripey tape that gave the place a feeling of visiting a crime scene. This tape must have been there to warn people that there was a pond and it must have been risk assessed as dangerous. The fields had barbed wire broken fencing, mostly lying on the ground. As we entered the main part of the house, the cold hit us. The house generally looked sad and uncared for and I actually felt sorry for the building. Despite the house and the land being badly neglected, we could see that the house must have been very grand in its time and we could see its potential. We wanted to look at the stables but to get to the stables we had to climb over the padlocked gates. The stables also looked neglected and worn. The whole place was dull and grey and there was no evidence of the happiness that the house must have known.

We decided that purchasing the house and land was worth the risk. We were aware that the restoration of the house and land would be hard work as it was a huge project. We were also aware that this may take longer because we both worked full time. We put an offer in through the estate agent and the offer got accepted. We had surveys completed but then we hit a problem, the bank accepted a higher offer from another person, apparently they can do that even though we had spent money on the surveys. This happened a couple of times more and we made our final offer, we were ready to walk away and to lose the money we had already spent if we were to be out bid again. This time the offer was accepted and the dream house was to become ours. We visited the house a few more times before we were given the keys so that we could get a better feel for the place. The land surrounding the house and the stables felt right for us but what we also loved was the abundance of wildlife. There were two ponds, a large one next to the stables and a smaller one next to the garage. The house and land was the home of a few Mallard ducks, Moorhens and Coots. There was a stream at the bottom of the garden with a small stone bridge which entered one of the fields. Everywhere you looked you could see signs of wildlife, the garden was a haven for rabbits. At night, there were bats, owls, foxes and badgers. As we walked down the drive on one of these visits early in December 2017, the light was fading in the late afternoon, a barn owl flew over our heads. The light caught the white underneath of the owl which reflected back at us. At that moment, I thought, 'Yes, we can make this our home and Mum will love it here too.'

We moved into the house later in that month on 17th December 2017, which was another good omen as it was Dad's birthday. He would have been 83 years old the day we moved in. We took an electrician and a plumber with us to check that the electricity was safe and that there were no water leaks when they were switched on. When houses are repossessed you hear of all sorts of vandalism that is carried out by the previous owners. I suppose the reason for this is partly grief for what they are losing and also anger for what is being taken away from them. We were given a large bag of keys which we had to identify as none of them were labelled. Andrew's sister, Alison, and his niece, Chloe, came along to help us to figure out which keys belonged to which lock, every key hole had three keys so this took us a while and we treated it like a game, dashing around the house to see who could identify the most keys. They stayed for the afternoon also helping us to clean the carpets. The first night we stayed at the house, Andrew managed to get the log burner roaring. We opened a bottle of wine to celebrate and sat down in the conservatory. We were so happy celebrating our first night in our new home in front of the cosy log burner. Unfortunately, this was when we found out that the conservatory roof leaked badly. Andrew had rain drops falling on his head. Andrew just looked up at the ceiling, stood up, left the room and returned wearing his Australian waterproof hat. He then sat back down again and with a smile made a toast to our new home. We were blissfully happy just being there and living in the moment. The next day when we tried to use the hob in the kitchen we soon realised that it had been vandalised, as well as all of the other kitchen appliances. We spent the first few months of living at the house, eating out every night and living off a carvery at the local Hotel Rudyard until we managed to replace all of the kitchen appliances.

During the first few weeks of living in the countryside it took a lot of getting used to because it was so noisy. You think that the countryside is quiet but this a false belief. At night the noise was incredibly loud. We seemed to be on the flight path of 200 plus Canadian Geese who were neighbours as they lived on the Mill Pond next door to our house. From December to February they fly over our house in the night several times, sometimes circling the house and garden and at other times flying directly over. It seems that they have a lot to say to each other whilst flying over. They make regular trips to Rudyard lake which is just down the road from where we live and then they return to the Mill Pond. They can't seem to decide where they want to be and so continually travel to and from the lake to the pond. They constantly honk and chatter to each other. At night it took me months to get used to the sound. In the day they sometimes used to land on our pond which created all sorts of chaos with the other birds that live there. They all seem to be arguing, it was very comical to observe and they didn't seem to care about us being there at all.

We were aware that there was a lot of work to do to the house, inside and outside as well as work to do on the land so we wrote a priority list which covered four pages of an A4 writing pad. It looked like an impossible amount of work that needed to happen. From the priority list we came up with a plan of action. The plan moving forward was to get the house sorted so it was fit to live in and then Mum could start coming to stay at the weekends. This would acclimatise her to the house whilst maintaining her independence for as long as possible. There was also a lot of work to do outside which was a bigger priority so that we could move our two horses, Aine and Basil to the house. All of the fencing was unsafe and broken with lots of barbed wire sticking out or lying on the floor. So that became our first outdoor priority. Our horses were living at a livery yard in Alsager. Full or part time livery is expensive and the livery yard was a good 45 minutes away. So if we could sort the fields and the fencing we could save money by not paying livery and we would also save on the fuel costs. Meanwhile keeping the horses in Alsager meant that I could call in to see Mum after l had seen to the horse's needs.

The previous house owners had fly tipped in a whole paddock, huge general rubbish bales which smelt badly of decay and was likely to attract vermin. When we first looked at this paddock, it looked like there was a large grass bank which was about 6 feet in height and spread across an area of approximately 20 x 10 metres. However, we soon realised that this grass bank was a mound of fly tip rubbish. We hired skips, donned a pair of gloves each and gradually started to clear out the rubbish by hand into wheelbarrows and then tipped it into a skip. This was a grim job and took several weeks of grafting to complete it at the weekend as well as 16 large skips. The rubbish included anything from an old bed with its mattress and springs, tin cans and dirty nappies. There was evidence of partially burnt rubbish as well as we dug deeper. We couldn't understand why someone would dump this rubbish on their own land. We came to the conclusion that the previous owners must have been paid to take the rubbish as one of the neighbouring farm properties also had bales of general waste dumped at their property. However, the neighbouring farm had a far worse problem than we did, they had hundreds of rubbish bales compared to our small paddock of waste. We concluded that the only reason for this neglectful act, on a property that would have been very grand and special in its time must have been desperation for money.

We contracted a local fencing company to remove the old barbed wire and broken fencing and replaced it with safe post and rail fencing. In total there was one kilometre of fencing to replace. We made the stables ready for our horses when the fields were safe and ready for them to come to live with us. We spent Christmas 2017 in the house but the kitchen was not ready so we joined Allister and his wife, Cathy at their home in Alsager with Mum for Christmas dinner. Not long after Christmas we got the house in a reasonable state so Mum could come and stay with us at the weekends. Mum's room was downstairs with easy access to the kitchen, it had a wet room and was very cosy. Mum loved it. It had patio doors which overlooked the garden. This part of the garden was popular with garden birds as well as rabbits and squirrels. We placed bird tables and feeders just outside of Mum's window so that she could watch the wildlife. Mum loved wild birds, well she just loved nature and any animals actually. We did the Great Backyard BBC bird count in February 2018 and counted an incredible amount of species of birds which even included a pheasant that lived in the garden whom we nicknamed Phil. Mum called her room "a room with a view".

Mum loved coming to stay at the weekend, she would wander down to the stables and help me with tack cleaning. I would wrap her up in a blanket and she would sit polishing the leather of the bridles. She could stroke the horses whenever she wanted. She loved our Border Collie cross dog who was called Elvis. He was 12 years old and showing his age but he loved Mum and enjoyed her company. Mum had always had Border Collies and she used to call him Robert who was her last Border Collie but he didn't seem to mind. Mum didn't seem to miss her own home, she was very happy to stay with us and the animals. She seemed to be more attached to me than she was to her home which made the transition very easy. She never asked to go home like Grandma used to, well not until much later as her dementia progressed. I would go to pick her up on a Friday evening after work, she would be ready with her bag packed waiting at the door. Mum would stay until Monday when I would drive her back to her home and on the way we would call at the shop to get her weekly groceries. Then for the rest of the week, Allister would call in every evening to see if she was ok. We had a routine going that seemed to work for everyone, although it did not leave Andrew and me with very much quality time together.

⋯⊷⊷◁▷⊶⊶⋯

Chapter 6

Juggling Act

Mum continued to visit us every weekend and this was working out quite well. However, Andrew and I didn't feel that we were getting any time for us. We have always been very close, insular in many ways as we are best friends. We work and do all of our hobbies together. Therefore, it felt quite challenging, even slightly claustrophobic, having to spend every weekend with another person. It sounds selfish but we missed "Our Time". Mum would watch television with us in the evening, she would rush into the front room for the best viewing seat but then she would complain that what we were watching was rubbish.

'What's this rubbish? Oh, I can't be doing with him!'

'Why don't you sit in your room Mum, and watch your television?'

'I want to be in here, with you.'

We would change the television station to something that interested Mum, only to find that after five minutes she had slumped in the chair with her chin on her chest, fast asleep and snoring lightly. Meanwhile, I would be sitting in the less comfy chair trying to view the television side on. I would give her a gentle shake to wake her so that I could ask her if she wanted to go to sleep in her room. She was adamant that she would not go to bed as it was too early and that if she went to bed this early she would not be able to sleep later. We gave in and listened to her gently snoring away. Living with other people can be difficult and even more so when someone has dementia. You know that they can't help it but irrational behaviour can really rattle you. When Mum eventually woke up she would then announce that she was going to bed. At this stage of her dementia, she could manage to get herself ready for bed independently. However, what she had started to do is list everything she was going to do to get ready for bed. She would say, 'Right, I'm going to have a strip wash, wash my face, wash my body and then...,' at this point my husband would be going a strange green colour and I would have to quickly interrupt her.

'We don't need to know all of the detail, Mum.'

'I'm not saying anything wrong, I'm just saying that I am going to wash down below and...'

'Enough, Mum, Andrew doesn't need to know all of the detail.'

She would then become slightly agitated and say,

'What's wrong with him? I was only going to say that I was going to wash my ...,' 'Stop it Mum!'

The same sketch would happen every evening. I could feel my brain anticipating this and it would make me anxious. Andrew is squeamish at the best of times.

It wasn't all bad though and it was really good to have Mum around for food preparation, we would cook and bake together. She was great at prepping the vegetables for dinner. She found that having me around to provide instruction gave her the confidence to help with the cooking. She used to love coming shopping with me and when her legs got tired she used to chat to people that she met whilst she rested on the chairs at the end of the aisle behind the checkout. Mum was a very sociable person and loved talking to people, she would then repeat the stories to me on the way home. Mum never wandered off whilst she was out shopping with me. Mum was also really useful in the garden and she used to help me with the garden pots. She loved to plant pansies and other flowers. There were lots of garden pots that Andrew had made out of old sherry and wine barrels dotted around the paths in the garden. There was an ornamental wishing well in the front garden. We planted herbs in some pots and flowers in others, the garden was brimming with colour. I used to take Mum to the local garden centre. Mum could remember a lot of plants even if her memory was fading in other areas. Mum and I had often bickered when Dad was alive but during this time we became very close. I think that was because she was with me all of the time.

In the early days of the weekend visits, Mum used to feel safe and content enough for us to leave her alone in the house for short periods of time. Horses need exercise and so most of my time is spent outdoors caring or training my horses. I enter competitions as well with my horses, competing in low level dressage competitions. Sometimes, Mum would come with us but if the weather was poor and it was not fit for her to come along, we would leave her alone in the house. Our dog, Elvis, used to keep her company whilst we were out. I used to write a note and stick it in a prominent place stating where we had gone. I would write my telephone number on the note so that if she forgot, she could look at the note to prompt her memory and if she needed me, she had my telephone number. Once whilst we were out one of our neighbours came to the house to sell tickets for a charity garden party. Mum looked through the window and tapped on the glass from the inside. She informed him that we had gone out and locked her in the house. She told him that she did not have a key to open the door. He left, very concerned and came back later when we were in and to check out Mum's story. When I asked Mum why she had told him that she was locked in she said, 'Oh, that strange man, that silly bugger, I don't know what he wanted, he was acting very strange.' I felt awful trying to explain to him that Mum was not locked in because I wasn't sure whether he believed me.

Frequently on our return from the horse show Mum would say,

'Oh thank goodness you are here, have you seen your father? He is late and I don't know where he is,' or 'I am looking for Alan, have you seen him?'

I found this extremely upsetting, the grief and pain that I suddenly felt in my chest was crushing me. I would have to compose myself, take a few deep breaths and then say,

' Do you remember what happened to Dad? Think back to what has happened, can you remember?'

Most of the time she would then slowly remember and become upset. She would start crying and berate herself for not remembering, it was heartbreaking. However, sometimes she would just complain that he was always late and messing in his shed. These re-runs of Dad's death would happen several times a week. I never became numb or unaffected to the devasting impact it had on my emotions. I wanted to shout, 'He's dead, stop asking me where he is,' but I had to remind myself that Mum didn't know he was dead so I had to be patient no matter how it hurt me. The best thing to do would be to try to distract Mum with a job to do. Once she was occupied with something to do, she was calmer and worried less.

As time went on, It became more and more difficult to leave Mum on her own. She developed a new obsession which was raiding the fridge to gorge on whatever food she could find. We decided that it was best policy to take Mum with us wherever we went. This took a bit of planning to ensure that wherever we went it was suitable for a person with a disability and that there was a suitable toilet that allowed enough space for me and Mum to occupy at the same time. There aren't disabled toilets everywhere. We would take Mum with us to the local dressage competitions which were held at Lodge Farm Equestrian Centre and Beaver Hall Equestrian Centre. I used to get my horse ready, then get Mum ready, then I would load Mum into the car, and finally I would load the horse into the horse trailer and off we would go. At Lodge Farm I used to take Mum to the toilet as soon as I got there. I would then help Mum to climb up the steps to the café. There was a viewing gallery in the café, the arena was inside so Mum could sit there and watch the horses perform. The young lady behind the counter knew Mum and would serve her Oatcakes with cheese filling and tea and then I would pay her afterwards. This was a great venue to take Mum, the staff there always kept an eye on Mum for me. Mum loved her Oatcakes, these are a Staffordshire savoury pancake which can be filled with different types of fillings. They are very different from the Scottish Oatcakes which are more like a savoury biscuit. We followed the same routine when going to Beaver Hall. The arena is outdoors there but if Mum sat by the window inside the cafe she could watch the dressage from the warmth of the cafe and on a fine warm day she could sit outside to watch. Mum didn't really understand what she was watching but she loved being out, people were so kind to her and they would spare a few minutes of their time to chat with her. On the return journey, we would come home, I would unload Mum first and then the horse. Many people manage to compete when they have babies or small children in tow and so we managed just like they do. I became very good at this juggling act.

At this point Mum was only coming to stay with us over the weekend. What I didn't realise is that when Mum was taken home on the Monday morning she craved more company. She would go visiting her neighbours or she would walk a good half mile to visit Thelma Bickerton. Mum always gave Thelma her full title out of respect. Thelma was a teacher at the school where Mum used to be the Caretaker. Mum was well known to everyone in her road as she had lived there for a long time. When Mum made these unannounced visits, the neighbours and Thelma were always welcoming and would offer Mum a cup of tea. She wouldn't just stay for a short while though, she would stay for hours. Mum was from the age where you didn't need to make an appointment to go visiting, you just turned up. In truth though she was overstaying her welcome but they didn't let on, they were just lovely kind people.

Our first winter in the new house was the winter of 2017/2018 and it was bitterly cold. On our return from work one day it was snowing. In Leek it can snow really heavily and we nearly didn't make it home from work due to five foot drift of snow in our lane. Our car at the time was a Land Rover Discovery and even with the 4 wheel drive it was struggling to get a grip. The snow was around for a week or so but that didn't put Mum off coming over. We kept the house warm with the log fire but we did need to keep going outside tending to the horses, making sure they were warm, fed and watered. Mum was under strict instructions not to come out of the house whilst I was down at the stables because the Indian stone path was extremely slippery. I was very worried that Mum may fall and hurt herself. Of course Mum paid no attention to these instructions and she would appear down at the stables but at least she was wrapped up well and used a Zimmer frame for support.

Spring 2017 soon arrived though and so we were able to recommence with the outside tidying up and jobs from the priority list. One of our tasks was to clear a field of Sycamore saplings. So, as soon as it was light enough to spend time outside in the evening, Andrew and myself could be seen in the field. We cleared approximately 500 sycamore samplings from the summer paddock which had managed to grow a few foot in height. We value trees and we have many on the land that line the fields and the brook that runs through the land. These saplings however, were never going to survive because they were too close together. The saplings had grown from seeds that had been scattered in the field by the wind from a nearby adult sycamore tree. They are also very poisonous to horses and so we had no choice but to pull them up. I have to say it was quite therapeutic. Looking back at the clear field and how many we had cleared was very rewarding. Fields and land need a lot of care and attention particularly if horses are kept on the land. Horses' hooves dig into the soil causing big holes, the horses congregate in areas next to gates which causes worn patches of grass. Fields need careful management including resting them. The care required includes harrowing, rolling and re-seeding if necessary. Fields can be overgrazed and grazing should be rotated. If the fields are not cared for then weeds can take over. It was obvious that the fields had not been cared for prior to our arrival and there was evidence of thousands of small Ragwort plants. Common Ragwort is a native biennial plant which grows to approximately 90cm with beautiful yellow flowers. Unfortunately, it is very poisonous to horses if they eat it as its toxic compounds cause liver failure. Horses won't eat this when it is growing unless they are starving but they will eat it if the plant is dead. The problem comes when there is that much of it, the horses have no choice but to eat it. Our fields were too risky to keep horses on as the Ragwort foliage was spread all over the ground. Andrew and I spent hours in the evening weed pulling, this kept us busy all week but we couldn't leave Mum for any length of time so weekend weed pulling was out of the question. We didn't want to use weed killer because of the harm it can do to other plants and insects. Being outside has always felt relaxing to me though, so I didn't mind.

Chapter 7

Basil, Elvis, Bowie, Mac and Aine

In March 2018, Elvis died, he was twelve years old. I had been working a night shift and had returned home at 6am. Andrew got up, we sorted the horses together and then Andrew took Elvis out for a walk around the field. On his return from the field, Elvis ate some left over steak for his breakfast. I went to bed and Andrew went to work. At 10am, I got up and Elvis was nowhere to be seen which was unusual for him as he always came to greet me. I went to look for him and found him in his bed lying on his side. He was dead and he must have died in his sleep. What a lovely way to go but we were both devastated and so was all of the family. He had been our boys' best friend when they were little and through their school years. He was an amazing dog, he had walked hundreds of miles with Andrew and me. Every year we used to complete a long distance walk with Elvis. He had walked the Pembrokeshire Coastal path, The Cleveland Way, Hadrian's Wall, The Cotswold Way, The Pennine Way to name a few. But the problem with animals is that we usually outlive them and when they are gone, there is a void. Andrew buried him in the garden and made a tomb around his grave. Mum was coming over the following day ready for her weekend visit. I wanted to tell her face to face rather than over the phone. When I told Mum she was also really upset. Mum had always been an animal lover. I remember when I was growing up that she had always taken in stray cats and any other animal that needed a home.

The following week the house seemed empty and it was quite frankly depressing. Every time we came home from work we were expecting Elvis to greet us. The house just didn't feel right without a dog and so after about a month we decided that we were going to get another dog. I had seen an advert for a Merle Border Collie that had been rescued and was looking for a good home. We thought it would be nice to rescue a dog rather than buying a puppy. I sent the local dog rescue centre a message on my phone, telling them that we were interested in adopting the Merle Border Collie. I explained that we were always outside, that we had approximately 15 acres of land and that we loved animals. Exercise was not a problem as we had lots of land and that we had always gone on walking holidays once a year with our previous dog. Border Collies need lots of exercise and I reassured them that we knew this as we were experienced with the breed. I soon got a reply and I was flabbergasted to have been turned down. They said we were unsuccessful because we work. We couldn't understand the decision and they didn't even come to see us to do a home check. They said that the dog would need to be in a home with no children, with people that didn't work and preferably who had another dog. It's no wonder so many dogs need re-homing is the conclusion we came to.

We were disappointed but we really wanted another Border Collie. The experience had put us off re-homing from a dog rescue charity, so we decided to buy a Border Collie puppy. I researched local breeders and found a responsible breeder who also checked us out thoroughly. The breeder said that she was expecting the litter to be born in May 2018. I told her that we wanted a boy and she agreed to reserve a boy if one was born. So that is how we ended up with Bowie who was born on 8th May 2018. Andrew and I went to see him when he was tiny and he fitted in Andrew's hand. Whilst we didn't have a dog, we took advantage of the time waiting for his arrival by cycling Land's End to John O'Groats (LEJOG). We didn't want to go on a walking holiday in 2018 without a dog, as we always called the walking trips "The dog's holiday". We did LEJOG cycle with Allister and two friends, Jen and Matt, and so we enlisted the grandchildren to take it in turns to call in on Mum and to take her to get her pension and shopping. Following the cycling, Bowie came to us when he was 13 weeks old. Bowie is a traditional black and white Border Collie with very symmetrical markings and a white stripe down his nose. Mum was over at ours ready for the puppy to arrive. For Mum and Bowie, it was love at first sight. What was to develop over the next couple of years was a very special bond between Bowie and Mum.

During the first eight months of Bowie's life he came to work with us and our staff used to take it in turns to take him for a short walk and toilet visit outside. This continued until Bowie started to chew through the Cat-5 cables at work. When he started doing this we found an amazing dog walking service called Perfect Paws which Bowie loved. Bowie was also taken to dog training once a week. He is a very friendly dog to all humans and dogs alike. We noticed that as Bowie started to grow he became very protective of Mum, he was assertive but not aggressive. He would sit in front of her or next to her for long periods and in return he got his ears tickled for hours and hours. As Mum became frail she needed to walk using a stick or a Zimmer frame. Wherever she went she took Bowie with her on his lead. She used to appear down at the stables with Bowie by her side. I was concerned that he was going to pull and unbalance her. However, he seemed to sense her vulnerability and he would never pull her. She would take him for short walks up the drive. If an unknown person came to the house, Bowie would go and sit at Mum's feet in between them and her. Michelle, the hairdresser used to come to do Mum's hair and Bowie would be there making sure that she was alright and that no-one was harming her. She wasn't always loyal to him though, she would often blame him for things that he was clearly innocent of such as eating ham that was supposed to be for a sandwich later. He didn't seem to mind though.

Frequently at the dining table I would see Mum throw food on to the floor. Bowie would snaffle up what was on offer. This is not something that we encourage because we didn't want a dog that begs all of the time plus we didn't want him to eat something that was poisonous to dogs. Try as I might, I could not stop her from throwing the food and she would just deny doing it. I would watch her like a hawk and she would watch me, both of us would pretend not to be watching each other. As soon as she thought I wasn't looking she would flick her fork and the food would fly through the air and onto the floor. Bowie was incredibly happy with the arrangement though and had no complaints.

'Stop throwing food on the floor, Mum.'

'I don't know what you mean.'

'Yes you do, just stop it, it's not good for Bowie.'

If either of us ever raised our voices at each other, Bowie would show his disapproval with a loud "Woof". He was Mum's protector but he would also tell Mum off with a "Woof" as if to say 'Enough, Stop.'

Border Collies have lots of distinctive traits and Bowie is no exception. He always wants to chase anything that moved which included fast jets and noisy motorcars. However, when he was with Mum, he was extremely disciplined. Bowie loves to chase light when he sees reflections and pounces on shadows like a Snow Fox. He entertained Mum and kept her occupied. His favourite place was sitting with his back to Mum so that she could tickle his ears. Tickling took precedence over everything else.

In the same year as losing Elvis, in August 2018; we also had bad news about my horse, Basil. He had been suffering for 6 years with a mysterious skin problem on his hind foot/leg in an area called the coronet band. This originally started when he had a tiny piece of thin wire stuck in his coronet band when he was 2 years old. The wire was removed in a surgical operation at the equine vets. At first the area healed but it would keep breaking out into an open wound, the surrounding skin kept becoming infected and eventually the coronet band started to split around his hoof. After 6 years of intense care and treatment, the vet decided that he needed an MRI scan at Leahurst Equine veterinary hospital. Our farrier, Russell came over to take Basil's shoe off ready for the MRI. We took Basil to the equine hospital in Liverpool where he stayed for a few days whilst they investigated, performed blood tests and the MRI scans. Andrew and I went along to receive the results and to have a consultation with the vet. We were looking forward and expecting to bring him home. However, the vet informed us that inside his foot was rotten and his hoof was only being held together by a thin structure within his hoof, he told us that at any time we could come home to find him in the field with his foot basically hanging off. The cause was likely to be cancer and there was no treatment. Basil never came home from Leahurst, we decided that it was kinder for him to be put to sleep. This was a dreadful decision to have to make especially as Basil was only 8 years old and extremely healthy in every other way. We always put the welfare of our animals first and we needed to consider the consequences of not doing anything. Basil must have been in a lot of pain. Horses are very good at hiding pain and will just carry on regardless of the pain that they feel. But, horses can't manage on three legs due their weight and Basil was a big horse weighing 700kg. We came home with an empty trailer and two broken hearts. Aine saw that the trailer was coming down the drive and she started calling and whickering for Basil. I phoned Russell to tell him that there was no need for him to return to replace the shoe. I had to clean out his stable and explain to Aine that her best friend wasn't coming home. I cried for days! The following couple of weeks were difficult as every time we went down to the stables to look after Aine, we were reminded that there was an empty stable. The veterinary hospital washed and plaited some of Basil's tail and mane, tied a blue ribbon to it and posted it to us which is now framed along with his last shoe. I needed to fill the gap that Basil had left in my heart and I couldn't bear to look at the empty stable. Also, horses are herd animals and need a companion. Russell, the farrier had a horse with a very similar personality to Basil and we often exchanged stories about Basil and his horse. Russell had recently stopped show jumping so I asked him if I could buy his horse, Mac. He discussed this with his wife, Zoe and after what seemed like an age, they agreed to let me buy him. Mac has an amazing and quirky personality. He loves to cuddle, kiss and have his bottom scratched. Mac patched up the hole in our hearts and has become Aine's companion.

Mac is a 17.1 hand high Belgium Warm Blood, bright bay gelding with very long legs and Aine is a 16.3 hand high, bay mare. Aine was nine years old when Bowie came to us and Mac was six years old. Aine is quite a sensible and gentle lady whereas Mac is playful with his gangly legs. Bowie was very curious with the horses especially Mac as he is the most reactive out of the two horses. When we first got Bowie we introduced him to horses slowly and carefully so as not to scare him. Aine will let Bowie sit next to her in the ménage and ignore him when he trying to round her up, like a working Collie. However, Mac is very playful. One day as we were walking through the horses' field Mac decided to play and chased Bowie across the field. Bowie was scared at first and then thrilled. Both Mac and Bowie have similar characteristics as in when they play, it escalates and then escalates some more. Neither of them has ever forgotten the field episode and they now they have the relationship where Bowie likes to stalk and chase Mac and in turn Mac loves to chase him. When Mum used to appear with her Zimmer frame with Bowie in tow, it amazed me that he never tried to chase either Mac or anything else that moved at speed. He knew that was not an option. He showed so much control.

Mac is my horse and Aine is Andrew's. We have a small arena at home to ride in so even when Mum was over I could ride without leaving Mum on her own entirely. When I ride Mac I have to be very careful as he is usually predictably unpredictable, he spooks at anything unfamiliar to his surroundings. This can be visual things, a strange noise or anything that has changed since the last time he saw it. Horses have small brains but parts of their brains are exceptional and memory is one of these parts. Mac will notice any subtle change to his environment and that can be a fence that has been painted or a bucket placed in a different spot to where it normally is. A spook is a startled jump sideways, or a quick change of direction with the intention to flee. Horses are flight animals and it is their natural instinct to run away from anything scary. This sudden movement can result in a rider's fall.

When Mum ventured outside, she always wore a hat. Mum had two favourite hats, one was a knitted white hat which looked like a Smurf or Elf hat and the other one was a bright light blue Trilby straw summer hat. Sometimes when I was riding Mac, I would hear Mum coming with the Zimmer frame. I would hear the scraping of the rubber bungs on the gravel path. Mum never picked up the Zimmer frame properly so it made a terrible grating noise. We had to keep buying spare rubber bungs for the bottom of the Zimmer because Mum would wear them out every few months. Mum is the only person I have ever known to wear out the bungs on the Zimmer. I would then glimpse up to see either a shock of white or blue. Then they would come into full view, Mum, the Zimmer, the hat and the Collie. OMG I would think, this is it, I'm going to be on the floor. I would shout trying to keep her at a safe distance, 'Go back to the house,' but she would keep coming a few steps further with the wheels now making a terrible sound of screeching as the gravel got stuck in the wheels preventing them from turning smoothly. Then Mum would decide to drag the Zimmer instead of rolling it.

'Go back to the house! Now!!'

Mum would look bewildered,

'But I just wanted to know if you had seen your Dad, I am looking for Alan.'

The bright blue hat was just visible behind a post which looked like a hat with no body. Mac would stand stock still trying to assess what he was seeing and hearing before spinning sideways and then Bowie would start barking to tell Mac off. We spun around with no control but I managed to stay on.

'Go back to the house! Now, please.'

Then the Zimmer would turn like Mum was doing a pirouette, small staccato steps until she was facing the opposite way and then the blue hat would go off in the opposite direction, heading back to the house. The sound carries where we live really easily as there is little to absorb it. I often wondered what the neighbours must have thought of me shouting for Mum to go back to the house with such a stern command.

One Sunday, I had entered a dressage competition at Lodge Farm Equestrian Centre. When we arrived, I took Mum to the toilet and then positioned her in her favourite place by the viewing window in the cafe. I asked the young lady behind the counter if she could get Mum whatever she wanted and top her up with tea. I would pay for anything that Mum had eaten and drunk after I had ridden. Once I was happy that Mum was sorted, I then tacked Mac up and started to warm him up. There were three more horses and riders to go ahead of me and then it was my turn. I had memorised my dressage test, Mac felt good and we were ready. One more to go and then me. Mum suddenly appeared at the entrance to the cafe and shouted across the warm up arena to me, 'Isabel, I need to go to the toilet, can you take me?' What was I to do, Mum couldn't wait otherwise she would be incontinent and if I took her I would miss my slot for the dressage. Just as I was about to get off and take Mum, one of my best friends arrived to watch me. We had known each other for thirty odd years, and luckily Jacqui is also a nurse. We did our nurse training together. Jacqui and Mum knew each other. Mum used to call Jacqui,

'Your daft mate.'

Suddenly it occurred to me that Jacqui could take Mum to the toilet.

'Jacqui, please can you take Mum to the toilet?'

'Are you sure she won't mind?'

'She won't care, she knows you.'

Relief! I thought all is good and I entered the arena for my turn in the competition. Dressage has very strict rules and etiquette such as no talking during your dressage test. There was no sign of Jacqui or Mum so they must still be in the toilet. I walked Mac around the arena once before the bell rang to say that I should start. Just as I was entering the arena, was when I became aware of the familiar screeching and rattling noise coming towards the arena. I knew instantly that the Zimmer was on its way back to the viewing gallery with Mum, Jacqui and the blue hat. The Zimmer frame rattled as it does when it is abused and the wheels screeched. Oh no, I thought, this is not what I need. As I came around the arena moving away from the judges' box I tried to speak as if I was a ventriloquist, 'Move back, move back, Jacqui sit Mum down and remove Mum's hat.' Bless her, Jacqui finally understood what I was getting at and got Mum to sit down just in time as I came around to that side of the arena. The judge was very considerate as well as I think she realised I was juggling with my responsibilities. Everything worked out well that day but it was really tricky trying to compete whilst Mum was with me, it was very distracting.

Sometimes, we would take Mum out for the day to the local garden centre which she enjoyed. We were limited in what we could all do because of Mum's limited mobility. On one occasion Andrew, Mum and I went along to a horse riding event as spectators. It was a One Day Eventing competition where a good friend of ours, Alison was riding. Eventing was first introduced as an equitation discipline to show the skills of the cavalry required for battle. Eventing consists of three disciplines which are dressage, jumping and then Cross Country. It became a sport in 1902 and was later introduced as an Olympic sport. At the higher more technical levels it is run over three days and at the lower levels can be completed in one day. Alison was competing in a one day event which is very physical for the horse and rider especially when you are an amateur. We watched the dressage and then the jumping. Mum was enjoying herself, I don't think she could really follow it but the sun was shining and she was having a nice day out. Somerford Park is where the event was and they put on a golf buggy to ferry spectators up and down the big hill. This meant that Mum could actually get on to the Cross Country course to watch. Alison was on the course and she went past so we all cheered her on. Alison, and Bertie her horse, completed the course, she looked exhausted, she was bright red and puffing. Mum said, 'That was great, is she going to go around again.' Mum used to make me laugh when she made such comments but it was clear that Alison would not be going around for another go. Mum was at her best when she was with other people, she used to make them laugh with her funny comments. Mum was very content when she was with Andrew and me. I am so lucky that Andrew accepted me, my horse obsession and my mother.

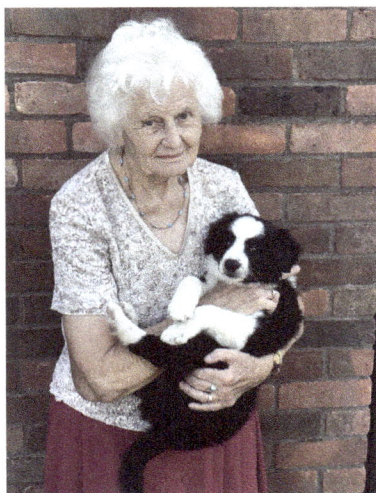

Mum and Bowie. Love at first sight

Chapter 8

The Strange Man

'*You can be in a room full of people, yet still feel alone.*' – *Quote of Unknown Origin.*

Mum had lived in Alsager all of her married life and she was well known by many, even more so because before her retirement she had been a Caretaker in one of the local primary schools. Whilst out walking in the village, she would stop and talk to people when she went shopping. Mum was very popular and had lots of friends who also lived in Alsager. Mum and Dad had always been the kind of people to help others and had a network of friends that they would visit. They had become close to their own General Practitioner and his wife. Saba was originally from Iraq, his wife, Gay was from Ireland. Mum and Dad had become very close to their family and their children looked towards Mum and Dad as grandparents. Dad did lots of DIY at their house and my parents took care of their dog when they went on holiday. They were always helping people and because of this they were loved and respected by many people in the village. When Mum was a Caretaker she became good friends with some of the teachers. She became particularly fond of a young teacher called Thelma and her husband, Anthony and their children. This friendship spanned over many years, beyond the time when Thelma had retired and her children had grown up. Mum used to walk around to their house and visit unannounced. She was always greeted and welcomed. When Thelma and Anthony's children had grown up, got married and had their own children, Mum would crochet blankets for the babies. These friendships were very important to Mum especially after Dad died. As the dementia took hold of Mum she would forget lots of people, however, she never forgot Thelma. Mum would visit Thelma more frequently and stay for longer. Thelma became a bit of obsession. I started to notice that Mum latched on to those around her that paid her a bit more attention. Thelma was one of these people, she was very kind to Mum. As the dementia progressed and as Mum became more confused, Mum would call me Thelma and I became Thelma in Mum's world.

Mum had six grandchildren of her own and eight great grandchildren. She had a special bond with the grandchildren. They would often visit her when she lived in Alsager. This helped Mum to live independently in Alsager because frequent visitors meant that there was always someone looking out for her. The idea was to get a rota of visitors to prevent Mum from being lonely. But Mum was lonely and had been ever since Dad had died. The dementia intensified her feeling of separation from him because they used to spend all of their time together. Mum was not attached to her house, she was attached to people and she loved having her family close by. Following Dad's death, Mum particularly became attached to me.

We continued to have Mum come to stay with us from Friday to Monday throughout 2018 and 2019. I would pick her up after work on a Friday and she would always be ready at the door with her bag packed, anticipating my arrival. If I was a few minutes late she would become anxious and phone me,

'What's happened? Is something wrong?'

'No, I'm on my way, just coming into Alsager now.'

'Oh, Ok, I thought something was wrong.'

She would be so pleased to see me and be happy all of the weekend when she was in our company. I would ask her what she had been doing in the week. She would tell me if she had been to visit anyone but she didn't tell me that she was constantly going from one neighbour and then moving on to another neighbour. A few months later, I found out that Mum was visiting her neighbours all day and she was basically constantly seeking out other people's company. The Strange Man would call to see her as well during this time. This was very concerning to me as I was worried about her vulnerability.

'What strange man? What did he want?'

'I don't know but he was acting really strange and then he asked me out on a date.'

'What did you say? What did he look like?'

'I told him I was married.'

I didn't know what to think of this, it seemed unlikely but I was worried. You never know who is around preying on the elderly.

When we got to our house, Mum would settle in and loved being with us. She wanted to be with me all of the time though. I was finding this attachment a little suffocating as she started to become more clingy. I would go out of the house to go to see the horses just for a break but five minutes later she would follow, wearing her blue straw or white Smurf hat. She loved wearing these hats. She always knew to dress up warm though. I have always been a person of independence and I like my own company. This attachment was very difficult for me to get used to and to rationalise. I had to adapt to having a follower so I would remember Grandma and how we would give her jobs. So when Mum appeared at the stables I would give her little tasks to complete. These included scrubbing horse feed buckets and tack cleaning. Mum became very good at cleaning tack, she would sit for hours cleaning and polishing until the leather was soft. My horses were very gentle with Mum. Aine appeared to be calm and understanding with Mum, she would lower her head and chew which is a sign that she was happy to be in the company of a person. However, Aine can get upset if a person is angry even if they are hiding it. I used to have a farrier to do her new shoes but this person was angry inside and must have emitted these emotions to Aine, so much so that she would become disturbed when he came to do her shoes, so I had to change to a different farrier. Aine was always calm with Mum and seemed to sense that she was vulnerable. Mac who can be boisterous was also calm with Mum, he loved a cuddle and he also liked to have his bottom tickled. Horses can sense vulnerability and that is why they make fantastic therapists. They are often used to help people with anxiety, depression, neurodiversity or post-traumatic stress disorder. This type of therapy involves spending time with horses which enables a subconscious positive effect on the brain that harnesses psychological and emotional benefits to a person. Horses have been used in Animal Assisted Therapy (AAT) since the early 1970s. Equine-facilitated psychotherapy is a therapy that involves interacting with horses which in turn helps patients to explore their feelings. Horses are very aware of emotional energies, horses sense what we're feeling, sometimes better than we do. Sometimes humans can hide their emotions from other humans with words and a forced smile. But humans cannot fool a horse. Horses can detect emotions that hide beneath the surface of our awareness and will often mirror them back to us. They can sense how you're feeling and what energies you are giving off. Horses have a calming influence, they can sense anxiety as well as understand breathing patterns. Horses have five senses like humans do but it is often said that a horse has a sixth sense. Horses are very intuitive animals and are much more sensitive than humans. Horses have always been my therapy; after a hard day at work I go to the horses and I can feel the stress evaporating. Mum would stroke the horses and they would respond in a very tender manner, my gelding Mac was particularly gentle with her. She had never had the desire to ride horses in her younger years but she adored being around them. However, Bowie was the one who had a special bond with her and he would become jealous if he saw her stroking the horses. We had to be careful that he didn't nip them. Being around animals was great for Mum, when she was with the horses or Bowie it had a positive effect on her mood and it seemed to calm her mind.

Whilst Mum was staying with us she wanted to make friends with our neighbours. She had met the neighbours who are closest in distance to our house on a number of occasions. We live quite remote so we only have one neighbour within walking distance for Mum's ability. Mum tried visiting the neighbour whilst we had nipped out, she managed to walk a few hundred feet to the end of our drive. She would take her trolley as this had a seat and she could put the brakes on it and sit down, where she waited for the neighbours to drive past. Mum craved company. She seemed to hate being alone. Sometimes, she would tell us that a strange man had come calling whilst we were out. The strange man started to make regular appearances but we never knew whether to believe her or not. The strange man scenario sounded very familiar. We had already had the experience of her telling one of our neighbours that we had locked her in but then more incidents started to occur. One day I walked outside to find a loaf of bread all broken up and thrown onto the patio area just outside the back door. I was concerned that we would get rats coming to eat the bread or that Bowie would eat it which would upset his stomach. When I questioned Mum about the bread and how it had got there, she said, 'Oh that wasn't me, it was that strange man, he started to throw bread over the hedge.' The hedge that she was describing is about 8 feet tall and on the other side of the hedge is a public footpath. The problem with this story is that although there is a public footpath along the side of the property, it is rarely used and it is unlikely that a person would be carrying a loaf of bread to throw over our hedge. We decided that she was making this up to cover up her mistake of throwing the bread away. The strange man quite often called when we were out whilst Mum was left on her own at our house. The strange man had called one day to ask Mum to go out for the day. On another occasion the strange man had called looking for Andrew and the strange man was wearing a big hat. We decided this was definitely not happening and that she must be making it up because she had been left alone and was feeling lonely or anxious. Then one day we bumped into a friend of ours who said that he had called last Saturday and my Mum had answered the door to say that we had gone out. He looked a bit puzzled when we asked if he was wearing a large hat. We felt a bit guilty that we hadn't believed her. Later on as the Alzheimer's progressed I mentioned the strange man to her Psychologist at the Memory Clinic and told him that I thought she was making up stories. He told me that it was possible that she was hallucinating. Mum may well have been seeing this strange man. Apparently, hallucinations are common for people with Alzheimer's to experience.

Another favourite for Mum was for her to repeatedly tell us that she was lost. We could see her anxiety levels rising if she was left on her own even for short periods of time. She would follow me down to the stables even when the weather was terrible and I worried about her falling. Quite often she would tell me that I needed to come in as the weather was turning bad, she would do anything to get me back to the house.

'Come on in, it's going black over Bill's mothers.'

I was used to this strange Staffordshire saying as I had heard it all of my life but Andrew was perplexed by it.

'It means that the sky is black over there and it looks like it is going to rain,' I would explain to him.

'No way! Who's Bill?'

'No one, it's just a saying that's from Stoke I think.'

It was so difficult dividing my time as I needed to care for my horses but I also needed to keep Mum safe. She just never wanted to be left alone. When she would suddenly appear, looking distressed she would say,

' Hello, can you help me? I'm lost.'

or her favourite was always,

'I'm looking for Alan, have you seen him?'

Her distress was awful to witness and I used to feel guilty for leaving her even for a short period of time. But when I needed to do other things, I just had to do them and hope that she didn't fall and that I would be able to calm her down later. When a relative has dementia, no one tells you how to manage it, there are no dementia workshops. However, there are a few books which say distraction is the best strategy. On a couple of occasions we went back to the Memory clinic for a medication review with the consultant. Mum was on the highest levels of medication to slow down the dementia and there was nothing else that could be done so she was discharged from the hospital outpatients. We were now solo with an unknown future to navigate as best as we could.

We continued with her weekend visits which were becoming progressively more difficult to manage. I would take Mum shopping on a Monday morning and then I would take her to her own home, in Alsager. Unbeknown to me, as soon as I had dropped her off she would go visiting to Thelma's or to one of the neighbours. The neighbours were very tolerant of her unannounced visits but she would quite often stay for hours. She would interrupt what they were doing and then stay for anything up to 3 hours, over staying her welcome. I only found this out after the start of the Covid pandemic when one of her neighbours called me to tell me what was happening and to raise a concern about breaking the Covid lockdown rules.

⚜

Chapter 9

The Covid-19 Impact

As a public health nurse I had been told by my college lecturer to expect a pandemic at some point. The World Health Organisation (WHO) had been predicting this event a long time before it happened. It was well known to public health professionals that a pandemic occurs approximately every seventy to eighty years. So when you look back at history we were well overdue for a pandemic. The last pandemic prior to Covid-19 was the Spanish Flu in 1918–1920. It was named the Spanish flu because it killed more Spanish people than any other nationality. The Spanish flu pandemic is still recorded as the deadliest pandemic in world history, infecting some 500 million people across the globe, roughly one-third of the population. The death rate was estimated anything from 17 million to 50 million, but some research estimated the numbers to be as high as 100 million. This was attributed to the movement of people during the first World War as well as general poor health. In recent years public health were concerned about bird flu and then swine flu thinking that they may be the cause of a pandemic, however, neither of these viruses reached pandemic status. The closest flu type illness to Covid-19 was SARS during the period of 2002 to 2010 and they mainly affected the population in China and Hong Kong. SARS stands for Severe Acute Respiratory Syndrome. In December 2019, we started to hear about another possible threat of a pandemic, it was called SARS CoV1 (Covid-19) and the outbreak was in China. It wasn't having any impact on the western world and everything carried on as normal. I remember watching the news and hearing about this strange virus which was spreading through China. The Chinese New Year fell on the 25th January 2020, this is a National holiday and many people travel abroad. This extensive travel meant that the virus also travelled worldwide and therefore this was the beginning of the pandemic. Although I had expected a pandemic and so had most public health professionals, what I had not expected was the impact of the virus and pandemic on the way we live and especially the restrictions that were to follow in order to contain its severity.

During the first quarter of the year we carried on as normal. We were hearing some scary stories but it all seemed a long way from the UK. We as a family continued with our routine of Mum coming to stay at the weekends and Allister keeping an eye on Mum midweek. In March 2020, Andrew and I decided to take a ski holiday to France. We asked Allister to keep an eye on Mum at the weekend. Going away is a massive logistical affair when you have horses and a dog even without an elderly dependant. We had to find someone to have Bowie for the week and someone to care for the horses. Aine stayed at home with someone coming to look after her, whilst Mac went to Wales for some dressage training to a friend's riding centre and Bowie went to stay with the dog walker.

We skied all week and had a great time. In the background we were aware that things were rapidly changing both in France as well as at home, the spread and impact of Covid was really fast and scary. People who had travelled back from China who had symptoms were being removed from their homes by men in white biocontainment suits. These positive pressure protective suits, are highly specialised, totally encapsulating, with an air fed breathing mask and are only usually seen in laboratory facilities. This must have been very scary for the people who were taken away and no one seemed to know where they had been taken. It was like watching something from a Science fiction horror film but this was real and playing out in front of us on the BBC news. There were lots of other scary events being shown over the next few weeks, buses loaded with passengers from China being taken to makeshift isolation facilities which were guarded. There were recommendations being made by the government to isolate everyone and to only allow essential contact.

Our business back in the UK started to feel the effects of Covid-19 whilst we were away on that ski holiday. The response was rapid as our clients started to cancel all of the work booked in for health surveillance in the workplace because they were told in a government recommendation only to allow essential visitors. The HSE stopped all health surveillance for workers as a way of reducing one to one contact. There was a feeling of mass hysteria which was building. Our business partner, Hayley was trying to keep things calm among our work colleagues as they were seeing all of their work being cancelled. This was leading our workers to worry about job security. All of our work more or less came to a halt over that week when we were away in France. Back in France we skied in the day but heard stories that there was a mass outbreak of Covid in a nearby ski resort. There was talk about shutting down all of France's ski resorts. In the day we skied and tried our very best to avoid other skiers especially on the chair lifts. We jumped on to one chair lift and at the last minute another person slid in beside me on the left. The lady was very friendly and chatty. I remember feeling very uncomfortable. It's strange how Covid was making us behave differently to other people.

'I have lost my friend,' she said.

'That's a shame, are you looking for her then?'

'Yes, she is Chinese and only flew in last night.'

OMG! I thought and quickly pulled my neck cover up over my mouth to resemble a mask and then I mimed for Andrew to do the same. I tried to shuffle to the right a bit farther and didn't make any further conversation. In the evening, in the hotel I started to plan for our return home and it was obvious that there were a lot of changes to be made both at work and at home. I paced backwards and forwards planning what needed to be done and what was a priority. It was beginning to look like our business could fail as a direct consequence of this pandemic. The day of our return finally arrived and as we flew back to the UK, we were told that France had indeed closed all of its ski resorts. The people that had just arrived were turned around to return to the UK. Looking at the news and what was going on, it became obvious that Mum could no longer stay in Alsager on her own. Lockdown was announced. I contacted my brother and asked him to look after Mum for another week after our return to England so that we could prepare for Mum to come and live with us permanently. We also needed to collect my horse, Mac, who was in Wales. Once we had collected Mac we needed a week to concentrate on what needed to be done at work.

Most people can remember March 2020, the start of Lockdown and the beginnings of a very strange period of time. Well, this was an exceptionally strange time for us! We landed in Manchester airport and everywhere had changed. People were wearing masks, staying two metres away from each other and I remember everyone treating everyone else with suspicion of being infected. How quickly and easily common courtesy and compassion can evaporate. On the way home we called into the supermarket to collect some essentials. I couldn't believe it, the supermarket shelves were bare. This was a total contrast to how the French people were reacting. We couldn't buy any bread, this had all been sold out. Home baking seemed to have become suddenly very popular, all of the flour and eggs had been wiped out. But trying to find any toilet paper was on a different level. People had gone mad buying lots of disinfectant and any other commodity that they envisaged they would need during a pandemic. The way that our supermarket work is Fast-Moving Consumer Goods (FMCG) that are supposed to be products on the shelves that sell quickly and are restocked quickly because of high consumer demand! However, the UK cannot cope with panic buying.

It was announced that travel was only allowed for essential reasons. We needed to collect Mac from Snowdonia where he was staying for training whilst we were on holiday. He was supposed to stay there for another week but we didn't know if things would become even stricter and we didn't want to risk him getting stuck in Wales. So our first priority on returning home was to rescue Mac. We were trying to work out whether we would be breaking the law but there were caveats in the guidance and it was not clear or concise. So the following morning, we set off for Wales with the horse trailer to collect him. I remember it feeling really eerie as we travelled down the A55 as it was empty. The A55 is usually a very busy main road from Chester through North Wales. As we were driving along, we wondered whether we were acting illegally, would this be classed as essential? It was my opinion it was alright as it was animal welfare. A police car came up behind us and I held my breath. What happens if he pulls us over and turns us around, how would we get Mac back? The police car just turned off at the next junction and I could breathe again. I was so relieved once we had collected him and we were heading home. We got home without incident.

The next priority was to reassure our work colleagues that we had a plan and a clear direction for the business. So the next day we went in to work to the office in Congleton. As we walked in, I could see about thirty four faces looking at us for leadership.

'Right, this is the plan,' I said, 'we are going to assess which office staff can work from home.'

I had been thinking about the plan for a week and in my head I had sorted out what was to happen on our return. We set about putting our emergency plan into place, we have always had this plan which covers emergencies but we had never had to use it before. I started to assess who could access their computers at home, confidentiality had to be considered as we deal with people's confidential medical data. The office staff dispersed with a plan of action for supporting our customers. Then we sent our technicians and nurses home to wait for further instruction; this gave us, the Directors, time to establish our next move. Our business is occupational health and if we couldn't help our clients now we may as well pack in the business. Our clients needed us more than ever especially as many of the companies are food manufacturers and classed as essential workers as well as FMCG companies. Our companies were faced with many obstacles to overcome and one of these was managing their staff when they had Covid-19 symptoms. The emergency health telephone lines such as 111 were completely blocked and you could wait for hours in a queue. The doctors' surgeries had shut. Our customers didn't know how to manage their workforce so we came up with a plan to help them. We set up a helpline which triaged our clients' employees when they were experiencing symptoms and directed them accordingly, providing health advice as well as indicating whether they were fit to work or not. This meant that their employees didn't need to try to access the NHS services unless they had an emergency.

Later on during the Covid-19 pandemic, our Occupational Health company was also one of the first approved companies to provide Covid-19 testing which helped many of our customers to remain open and functioning, especially those in manufacturing or the food industry. We also conducted respiratory qualitative face fit testing for first line workers such as the police, community staff and health visitors to ensure that their respiratory protection was working. If the masks didn't create a sufficient seal it would put them at risk so we played an important role in keeping these workers safe. Much later on in the pandemic when the Covid vaccine was developed we helped to vaccinate hospital staff on the Wirral. Our staff were amazing and they really showed that they were willing to adapt and eager to help others.

Going back to that first week following our return from France, once we had sorted out the horses and work, my attention turned to Mum and my Aunty Pam. Mum and Aunty Pam were cousins, they were both elderly and extremely vulnerable. However, they were also resilient to hardship, both had been children during the war and they had a tough British can-do attitude. Mum couldn't understand what was going on but she was aware enough to know that it was serious and was causing a lot of deaths. Aunty Pam was wise and knew everything of what was playing out around her, however, she could not comprehend what was going on with the panic buying in the supermarkets. She told me about a nurse whom she had seen on the evening news crying because she had come off shift only to find out that there was no food on the shelves when she went shopping. The evening news became an essential watch for us through the pandemic and we watched it avidly every night. It was the main place where information was shared about the fast changing rules about what you could and couldn't do. The government had a panel of experts who addressed the nation most days laying out the rules for us to follow. It was an unprecedented time, the government were faced with something that they didn't seem to have a clear plan for and so the rules and advice kept changing. I suppose they were trying to balance the scales of stopping the Covid transmission whilst also trying to keep the economy going.

One piece of advice was that people should not visit elderly relatives due to the risk of passing on the highly infectious Covid virus and that the elderly and vulnerable should stay at home. The advice was for the vulnerable people to shop online which meant that online supermarket shopping slots became very difficult to obtain and the slots were at a premium. It was recommended that the elderly had shopping delivered by friends, relatives or volunteers to the doorstep and left there rather than going in to the property. This was not going to be possible with Mum as she didn't understand social distancing or a ban on visiting. The time therefore seemed right for Mum to come and live with us and we were prepared because Mum had been coming over at the weekends anyway. When I arrived at her house to pick her up, the neighbours came over to the car and told me of their concerns because Mum had just continued to visit them regardless of the new strict isolation rules in place. They were worried that they were going to be in trouble for breaking the law by letting her into their house but they didn't want to turn her away. Quite a few neighbours came out of their doors to give Mum a wave goodbye as they knew that she was coming to live with me permanently. There were a lot of scared people and this showed on some of their faces. Mum appeared to be very happy to come to live with Andrew and me, she never showed any hesitation and she didn't appear to be sad about leaving everything behind. I did take quite a few of her favourite possessions so that her room in our house felt more homely and familiar.

Aunty Pam is my second cousin rather than an aunty but she had always been Aunty Pam to me. Aunty Pam's husband, Uncle Sam had died of lung cancer, the same year as my Dad in 2016. Since then I had either taken Pam shopping or I had done her shopping on a weekly basis and I still do, she is now 92 years old. I manage her finances, take her to hospital when she has an outpatients appointment and generally take care of her when she needed me to. She continues to live independently. Aunty Pam was born in 1932 and was three years older than Mum, they had always been close friends as well as cousins. Aunty Pam is bright as a button with all of her faculties, she still does crosswords and word searches, she has a great sense of humour and she is quick-witted. However, her body at the time of the pandemic was failing her and she could no longer walk unaided. She is a very sociable person who loves having someone to talk to. All of a sudden during the pandemic, Aunty Pam had no visitors due to 'Lockdown' and she was already lonely before but now she was also isolated. I decided that I could not just leave her food on the doorstep due to her mental well-being, therefore, I decided to create a bubble between her, me and Mum. I carried on visiting her once a week and for quite a while I was the only person she saw. Sometimes, I used to take Mum with me but I was always very careful that we were symptom free. Mum and me were the only people that Aunty Pam saw for months. Neither Mum or Aunty Pam appreciated the problem with empty shelves and food shortage in the supermarkets. Food such as yogurts were being rationed. Aunty Pam was very fussy on the size of the tomatoes or potatoes that she wanted. She used to complain to me that I had not brought her the correct food, the tomatoes didn't fit into the palm of her hand, I had got the wrong brand of toilet roll or that the bread slices were too thick. You would think that people who had lived through the second world war would be better at accepting rations but they definitely weren't. I think she used to expect me to get things off the black market like they did in the war. Mum could not understand why she wasn't allowed to visit people anymore or what was going on. One day I took her for a short drive through Alsager town centre to show her how deserted the roads were and how the people who were out wore masks.

Mum did settle into her new home though really quickly and seemed very content living with us. I think she quite liked the fact that there was a 'Lockdown', we had nowhere to go at the weekends and so she had plenty of company. Mum particularly loved the nature that was living in our garden, in the fields and generally around the house. The pond was always a hive of activity especially during the spring time. We had noticed that every year, two Canadian Geese build a nest on the island in the middle of the pond. The female would sit on the eggs for approximately 28 days, only coming off them to stretch her legs and have a short swim before returning to the nest whilst the male would swim around and wait patiently for the birth of the goslings. During lockdown we noticed so much wildlife, I wondered whether this was because we recalibrated and took the time to notice what was around us. I wasn't sure whether I noticed more wildlife because I was doing less so had more time to notice or whether the wildlife was enjoying Lockdown as life seemed quieter on the roads and in the towns. We live in quite a remote area which has the advantage of living amongst the wildlife and feeling part of that world but the downside of trying to work in a remote area is that we did not have good internet connection. So we had to go out and travel to work each week day. As we were classed as essential workers we were allowed to travel to and from work. We would leave Mum with Bowie and go to work in the morning. I was concerned at first with Mum's dementia but she seemed quite at ease. She never tried to leave and Bowie was good company for her. However, she did try to walk to the neighbour's house on a couple of occasions but she soon gave up on that idea as the drive is very long and uneven. Mum walked with a Zimmer frame or a blue mobility walker. If she took the mobility walker, she could walk farther and she could rest for a while when she was tired because it had a seat. She enjoyed wheeling up the drive, sit down and watch the cars go by. She would take Bowie on his lead and she seemed very content to be living with us at our house.

Mum was always pleased to see us return from work each evening, she would greet us at the door with Bowie. In the evening she would help me to prepare for our evening meal. The evenings were always the worse for Mum as she seemed to get very confused at night. Mum would constantly ask where Dad was and she would berate him for going missing again especially when he wasn't there for his meals.

'Where is Alan? He knows what time his tea is, where is he?'

I would have to repeatedly try to remind Mum that Dad wasn't coming home for his tea. This caused me a lot of emotional pain to relive the death of Dad over and over again. She forgot every night that he had died and I used to have to jog her memory by asking her to remember what had happened to Dad. She would say, ' Is he dead? oh no,' and then she would burst into tears.

We didn't really have any neighbours that we could see from our house but during 'Lockdown' we went outside every week like so many others to clap for the NHS. On the 5th July 2020, we could just about hear our neighbours clapping as well. Mum was clapping away and calling Bowie, I took a short video and Mum looks so happy on it. Mum clapped with us and she was smiling away, along with the nation who were also showing their appreciation to the doctors, nurses and care staff working in such an arduous time. The images of the nurses and doctors working in the hospital with air-fed masks on and scrubs was heart felt. They really did a great job and their best in such unprecedented times. The death toll kept rising and Covid was taking the lives of healthy young people as well as the vulnerable and the old. The number of deaths were announced every evening on the television.

Unless you were a key worker, you weren't allowed to work. However, people needed to work to pay their bills and for essentials such as food. The government came up with a staff retention scheme they called furlough. Furlough was designed to keep people's jobs open whilst they weren't allowed to work and to help the economy so that there was still a workforce once the pandemic was over. The government paid for 80% of their wage whilst they stayed at home. This provided enough money for people to live on. A lot of people were furloughed during 2020 at the height of the pandemic. We furloughed some of our staff but only for a few weeks. Once our company had started Face Fit testing, Covid testing in factories and later on, some of our nurses assisted with the Covid vaccination program there was no need to have people on furlough. All of our staff were busy and classed as essential workers. Andrew and I were also classed as key workers and we were extremely busy at work during this time. We did get used to seeing only a few people and we loved our time spent at home. A lot of people reassessed their life during this time as it gave people an opportunity to reflect. My priority was to keep Mum and Aunty Pam safe as well as keeping the business running smoothly. It was an incredibly challenging time but working with Andrew, pulling together as a family, enjoying my horses and Bowie helped me to stay mentally strong during this time.

Chapter 10

The Carers

Mum had always been a 'Faller' for as long as I can remember. She would fall over and get bruised, get up and brush herself down and then carry on with what she was doing. Dad used to say, 'That woman has bones like a horse.' When she was younger she had been hit by a motorbike that was speeding through the village whilst she was crossing the road. She was flipped up into the air to the height of about six feet and landed heavily. She was conscious but unable to move her legs so she was rushed to hospital. When they X-rayed her all of bones were intact but she had severe bruising and had developed a deep vein thrombosis in her left leg. She had to spend a week in hospital. Dad concluded that if you could survive that type of accident without breaking a bone, she was unlikely to break a bone falling over in the garden.

Ashley is one of our grown up children who works as a senior manager for our company. He normally lives in London but he had come home due to the Covid-19 pandemic as London was deemed to be unsafe due to its huge population. London was definitely not the best place to be, if you were trying to avoid the virus. At this time we still did not have sufficient WiFi connection at home so Andrew, Ashley and I went to work as usual. Mum stayed at home with Bowie. The three of us returned home from work one day to find Mum lying on the floor in the conservatory. She was lying there quietly until she tried to move and then she was screaming in agony. Bowie was sitting next to her looking very concerned.

We don't know how long she had been lying on the floor but it was obvious that Bowie had not left her side. Mum told us that she had been walking without her Zimmer frame. Sometimes, she did this and did what I call furniture surfing. Whether she had lost balance or slipped on a patch of wet flooring due to the conservatory leaking, we will never know. I asked her whether she had tripped over Bowie and she told me she hadn't. This fall was during the pandemic Lockdown and getting any help or an ambulance was near to impossible. We tried to get Mum off the floor but she was screaming. I ran upstairs and got a large bath towel, we put it behind her and gently the three of us managed to lift her into a chair. Mum's colour was normal so I didn't suspect shock. However, Mum told me that her upper left arm was extremely painful. I had a feel of it and thought it was alright, maybe badly bruised. I never for a minute imagined that her arm was broken, however, just to be on the safe side I thought it was best to take her for an X-ray. The problem was, where to take her? The BBC news was full of stories of people dying in hospital and the Accident & Emergency (A&E) departments being overwhelmed with Covid patients. Mum was elderly and she was more vulnerable so taking her to the main hospital in Stoke-on-Trent was a major risk. One of my friends and fellow nursing colleagues, Alison, whom I had completed my nurse training with as well as worked with thirty six years earlier was a matron in the A&E department in Stoke. The Royal Stoke University hospital was the nearest main large hospital to where we live. I telephoned Alison to ask her what the state of affairs was at the hospital with the Covid crisis. She told me, 'Do not come here, it's too dangerous for your Mum due to the risk of her contracting Covid.' Alison informed me that at the Royal Stoke, they had one entrance for non-Covid symptom accident and emergencies and one for people with Covid symptoms but she still believed it to be unsafe. Alison told me to take Mum to a smaller peripheral hospital called the Haywood hospital as she thought it was safer. There were no ambulances available during this time for this type of injury and the wait for ambulances was extensive anyway. So we bundled Mum into my car which was extremely painful for her but she put on a brave face and I took her to the small local hospital. We sat waiting our turn, wearing our masks, Mum looked very pale and exhausted. After a few hours Mum was sent for an X-ray and we were eventually seen. Mum had sustained a clean and complete break of her left humerus bone in her upper arm. I couldn't quite believe how bad the break was when I looked at the X-ray which was shown to us both. I don't know how she was managing with the pain. She was seen by a senior nurse and provided with a collar and cuff sling, prescribed strong analgesia and then we went home.

This presented a whole new challenge with regards to work. Mum could no longer stay at home on her own until her arm was healed. She would not be able to take herself to the toilet or make herself any drinks or food. She would also be unsafe when trying to mobilise with her Zimmer frame as she really needed both hands. Mum needed full time care but I really needed to go to work as the business needed my expertise and leadership especially during the Covid crisis. We had approximately thirty six members of staff relying on us for support and leadership and it was a very frightening time to be working. Our staff were helping front line workers to stay safe so it was vital that I attend work. I didn't know what to do about Mum as I also needed to keep Mum safe from Covid. Mum was my number one priority but when you have other responsibilities you can't just walk away from them. I was also aware that if I used a care agency who provide carers, they would be going into nursing homes which were all over the news as places of high contamination of Covid. Even if they weren't going into nursing homes or the hospitals, they would be going from one person's home and then on to another and another, thus increasing the risk of Mum contracting Covid when it was at its most deadly. A lot of the carers working for the agencies just didn't have sufficient training in infection control and they didn't have access to the PPE or equipment to deal with infection control at this high risk level. PPE had become very difficult to obtain and most of what was available was allocated to the NHS hospitals. There were stories of carers in nursing homes having to use bin bags as aprons during this time. We found out later that the government had sent a lot of our national PPE stock to China to help them which left us short. In our company we also needed PPE for our staff. When we tried to buy PPE, it was hard to find but when we did find some for sale, the companies selling it had quadrupled the price. A simple FFP3 mask which would normally cost £6 was escalated to the cost of £26 each and a pack of 100 very thin aprons which would normally cost pennies each were being sold for £25. The PPE companies were cashing in on this pandemic, there was a monopoly and there was nothing we could do about it, we just had to buy it. This inflation of PPE goods was disgraceful in such a time of need.

Hospital Covid patients were being discharged directly into nursing homes and I knew that was really dangerous to the residents. I knew that I didn't want carers to come to care for Mum who were going to visit lots of other people. Then I had a thought. One of my horse acquaintances and a relatively new friend called Sharon was a self-employed domestic cleaner. Sharon had suffered what a lot of people did at the beginning of Covid by having all of her work cancelled. People were being urged not to mix with other people and this included having cleaners come to your home. So I had a light bulb moment, I phoned Sharon to ask her whether she would like a job that paid the same as what she got for cleaning. I asked her whether she would consider coming to sit with my Mum and to keep her company. I told her that I only expected Mum to need the help for approximately six weeks until her arm had healed. Sharon immediately agreed to do this as it would help her out too as she was suddenly faced with no income means. At that time, Mum didn't really need any nursing care, she just needed some help walking to the toilet, getting food and a companion. This suited Sharon as she did not have any carer experience. I explained what the job entailed which would include helping Mum to walk to the toilet, helping her with her clothes, preparing her some food and giving her plenty cups of tea. Sharon would be there to generally just keep Mum safe.

Sharon started work as a carer the next day at 08.30 hours. This meant that I could go to work without worrying about Mum. So this was the beginning of a long term relationship between Sharon and Mum. Sharon was a bubbly person with a can-do attitude, she was kind and had patience with Mum. Mum's arm healed well and quite quickly and she was discharged from the hospital care after a six week review at the fracture clinic. However, the fall had taken a toll on Mum's health, it had knocked her confidence and it had accelerated the dementia. It was clear that Mum now needed permanent care and could never be left alone for long periods of time. We would never be able to leave Mum alone for eight hours whilst we went to work. What became obvious is that the fall and the trauma of the broken arm had exacerbated the Alzheimer's dementia. The change was substantial and incredibly quick. Mum had become vastly more forgetful and confused. She also became very clingy especially to me and she would worry when I was going outside to the horses. She also started to struggle with activities of daily living such as washing and dressing. I now had to do everything for Mum with regards to her personal hygiene. In the morning I would get up, rush out to go and feed the horses, then I would rush back inside to wash and dress Mum, prepare and give Mum her breakfast and then rush back out to Mac and Aine to muck out and then to turn them out into the field. Sharon would arrive at 8.30am so I could leave for work. I would work all day and then return at 5.00pm to relieve Sharon of her duties. We had this routine sorted. Sharon was with Mum all day, Tuesday to Friday and I was then Mum's sole carer on a Monday and every night.

Following the broken arm, the hospital referred Mum to the Falls Team which is standard practice following an elderly person falling. The idea is that the Falls Team made up of Occupational Therapists and Social Workers come out to assess the home in order to try to prevent further falls. The Occupational Therapist Team came out to assess our house. Following this assessment someone arrived to erect a step with handles just outside the front door which was bolted to the floor. This was an ugly contraption but necessary to prevent Mum from falling especially as our doorstep is quite high and goes directly onto slippery Indian stone. A commode was provided for emergencies and a new more stable Zimmer frame was given to Mum. The Social Worker said Mum could have prescribed incontinence pads which was really beneficial because they were better quality than the ones you can buy in the supermarkets and they were a great cost saving. These aids were received with gratitude and it was good to know that I could call the Occupational Therapist team if there were further aids that we needed.

Sharon agreed to stay on past the six weeks and so we got settled into the new routine. With Sharon on board it was a big relief to know that someone was with Mum in the daytime. Sharon and Mum would do jigsaws or colouring in Mum's adult colouring book. Mum would fall asleep a lot and so Sharon took on my cleaning to prevent her from becoming bored. Mum was very content knowing that someone was there all of the time. Mum continued to look for Alan and she repeatedly asked where I was but she was easily distracted. Sharon had Mum laughing at lots of things and they got on really well. When we got home from work every evening, Sharon would need to leave straight away to go and sort her horses out and to get back to her dogs. Therefore, Mum had to be left alone in the house for an hour whilst I would go out to sort our horses and then come back in to cook dinner. After dinner I would assist Mum to have a wash or give her a shower, get her ready for bed and then settle her down to watch television. After such high pressured days at work, I really looked forward to a relaxing evening in front of the television. The days started at 05.30am and work was full on and mentally taxing every day during the pandemic. However, in the evening Mum had other ideas and plans for us which did not include relaxing. In the early days of Mum living with us, she used to sit in the lounge where our television is set up but we had to stop that because she never wanted to watch what we wanted to. She would claim the best seat in the lounge and then constantly complain about what we were watching on the television.

'What's this rubbish on the television?'

'It's a programme that we like Mum.'

'Well I have never seen such rubbish.'

Sometimes, Andrew tried to enjoy a football match, he is an avid Liverpool fan and does not appreciate interruptions. Mum would make negative comments about his beloved team. These negative comments made me feel tense because I knew it would be annoying Andrew. He tried his best to be patient but he found this general criticism of anything that we were watching draining and frustrating.

So, we got Mum her own television for her bedroom so she could watch Coronation Street or a Question of Sport. Mum would watch the television for a short period of time, maybe half an hour but then she would start wandering. I was worried that she was going to fall again and so I would get up and go to escort her back to her room. One night I counted getting up from the sofa to go to see to Mum thirty odd times during a film we were watching. We would hear her wandering, press pause, I would go to see what she was doing and settle her down again. Five to ten minutes later we would hear her wandering again and we would pause the film and repeat this cycle over and over again. It was very hard to follow anything on the television. There is nothing quite like the noise of a Zimmer frame rattling whilst it is being dragged and slid along the floor to grate on your nerve endings. Sometimes, Mum would try to move stealthily like but she never really managed it. I would go to see what she was doing and she would frequently say, 'I'm looking for Alan, have you seen him?' I replied, 'I am going to write a book and call it, "I'm looking for Alan".' This constant disruptive behaviour continued until it was time for me and Andrew to go to bed. At about 10.00pm I would make Mum a malty drink, give her a couple of biscuits as well as her prescribed medication. Mum was taking a cocktail of tablets to try to slow down the Alzheimer's but I don't think it was helping. The problem is how can you tell if it's working as there is no magic cure and you certainly would try anything to try to slow the dementia. I often wondered if this was actually slowing down the dementia or whether without the medication she would be the same. Following the snack and medication, I would escort Mum to the bathroom to brush her teeth and help her to go to the toilet before settling her down for the night. She had to be prompted to do everything at this stage but with a prompt she could still do most of her own self-care. Andrew and I would then go to bed, hoping for a restful night's sleep. Mum would get up in the night to go to the toilet and she seemed to manage this on her own, probably because she was now familiar with her surroundings.

At our house, Mum's bedroom was on the ground floor next to the hallway and opposite the kitchen. It was a beautiful room with turquoise wall paper with white flowers on and it had a view of the garden through double patio doors. We hung bird feeders just outside the windows and she could watch the wild birds as well as the cheeky squirrels eating the bird feed. She had a single bed and an antique chair next to it that we had brought from her own house. Mum loved her chair and said that she found it extremely comfortable. However, Mum did not like her bed and would not sleep in the bed for whatever reason that I could not work out. I thought it may be fear of falling so I purchased a cot side but she just refused to get into bed so she slept in her favourite chair. Her head was supported with a pillow, she had a blanket covering her body and her feet were raised on a foot stool with another pillow under her knees. She insisted that she was comfortable and so that is the way it was. Unfortunately, this meant that Mum could mobilise more easily and this is when she started to wander at night. We would hear her crashing around the kitchen and this would rouse us from our sleep. Bowie wasn't getting any rest either. This would happen frequently during the night, every night and we were worried that she was going to fall again. Andrew purchased a magnetic door alarm which was connected to the kitchen door and when the magnet was broken it played a Christmas ringtone which sang out next to my side of the bed. When she wandered out of her room and into the kitchen, the alarm tune would play, 'Let it snow, Let it snow, Let it snow'. Mum would leave her bedroom and enter the kitchen approximately every two hours. This would trigger the alarm;

Oh the weather outside is frightful,

But the fire inside is so delightful,

And since we have no place to go,

Let it snow, Let it snow, Let it snow

I was like one of Pavlov's dogs and eventually my feet were moving before I was even awake. As soon as the music started I was on my way downstairs in order to prevent a fridge raid or a fall. Sometimes I would find her creeping along and trying to open the door quietly, she had no idea that it was alarmed when it opened. She was very deaf without her hearing aids which she took out at night. She must have wondered how I knew she was on the move. I would escort her back to her room, give her a drink and a snack, help her to go to the toilet, cover her back up and then I would go back to bed. This would occur approximately every two hours through the night, every night. Then at 05.30am, my alarm would go off and we would begin another day of the same routine. It was just like the film Groundhog Day.

The weekends had started to become unmanageable as Mum started to deteriorate. She wouldn't stay in the house when I needed to see to the horses. She would wander out to find me and this was dangerous as the flag stones outside of the house can be slippery. Mum was becoming even more clingy and I felt like I was suffocating. I was tired and irritable. I needed more help so I put out an advert on Facebook for a carer to come to help me at the weekends. I interviewed and accepted two ladies for the job, they would look after Mum 8.30am until 4.30pm on alternative Saturdays and Sundays. This was a game changer for me as it meant that I could spend time outside and particularly with my horses without worrying about Mum. Debbie came from a recommendation from a friend and she was an experienced carer. Debbie was a quiet, patient and spiritual lady who would sit with Mum quietly and had a very calming influence on Mum. Karen had never worked as a carer before but she loved arts and crafts. She would spend time colouring, drawing and doing crafts with Mum. They even made an England banner for the world cup and Karen took a photo of Mum proudly holding the banner. She also got Mum crocheting again. Karen had never been able to crochet herself but she went away and learnt so that she could help Mum. Karen was also kind and caring. Sharon, Debbie and Karen would also do Jigsaws with Mum. Prior to the Alzheimer's, Mum used to love Jigsaws but as time passed she became more of an observer than a participating Jigsaw assembler. She still got lots of pleasure from sitting there looking at the pieces and trying to make them fit. The network of carers kept me sane, they were my lifeline to some normality. I will be forever grateful that they were there when Mum and I needed that support especially as there was no other support available. Prior to Covid there was a café in Leek that had a coffee morning for people to attend that had Alzheimer's but also where their relatives and carers could support each other. I remember watching the news one evening and there was an elderly couple on the news, he was the carer and his wife had Alzheimer's. He was trying to manage to care for her and to help her stay safe with no external help whatsoever. He was crying which made me cry as I understood how difficult it must be for him. He was desperately trying to care for his wife and trying to keep her at home with him. He was doing this through a pandemic when there was no help available to him. I felt that I really understood how difficult it was for him. It made me realise that however difficult it was for me, there were people out there with less support than I had. I had a supportive husband and a trio of caring people to help me in the daytime.

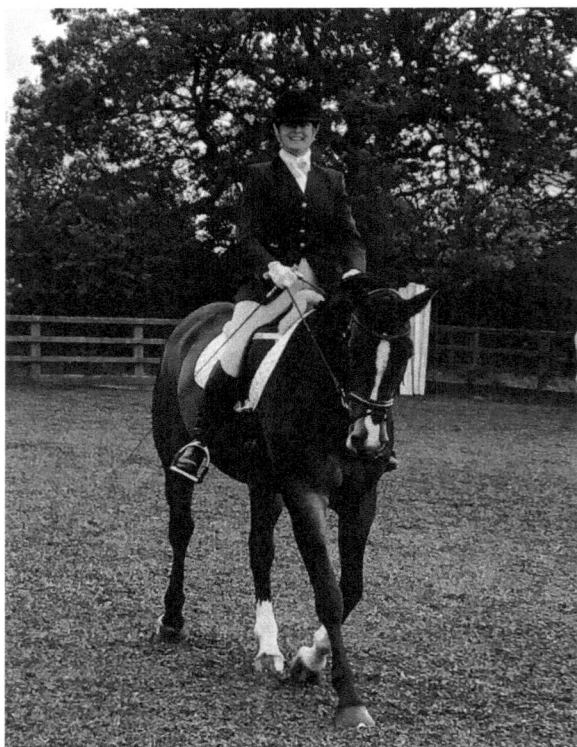

Aine and I competing at dressage at Alsager Equestrian Centre

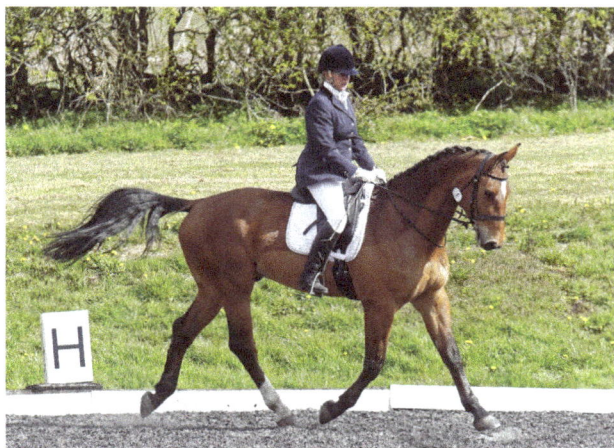

Mac and I competing at dressage at Beaver Hall Equestrian Centre

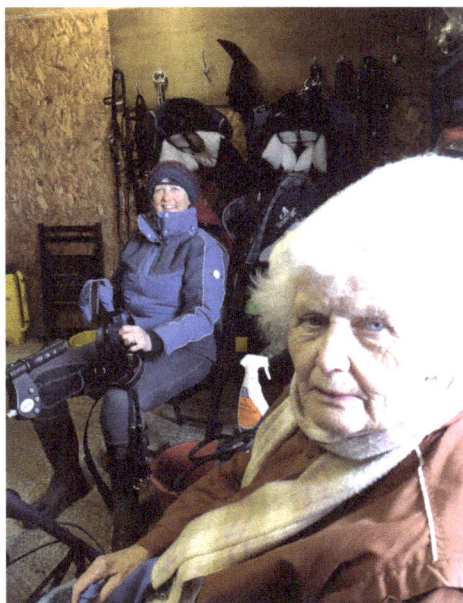

A session of tack cleaning

Chapter 11

The Fridge Raider

Mum began to develop an obsession with food. When I looked back into Mum's younger years she had always had a battle keeping her weight down. Like many women, Mum was very slim until she was pregnant with my brother. During the pregnancy and following his birth she had put on a lot of weight. This can be seen in old photographs, then I was born four years later and Mum's weight had increased again. Mum was determined to do something about her excessive weight and so she joined a slimming club. When I was young, I remember her dieting and this struggle with weight continued for most of her life. Her diet of choice was Weight Watchers and she was very proud to reach her target weight and received a medal for doing so. Mum managed to keep her weight in check but she remained on a reduced calorie diet for as long as I can remember. I don't know if this was an explanation for the food obsession and the strange relationship that she developed with food. She started with what Andrew and I called 'Fridge Raiding'. Mum would go into the kitchen and open the fridge every hour or so to help herself to food. This was not really a problem to begin with but sometimes she would eat what I intended to cook for dinner or anything else she may have found.

The fridge raiding was worse when I left her alone such as when I popped out to go down to the stables to the horses or when I was busy doing something. Being left alone was definitely a trigger. Mum gorged on whatever she found edible and sometimes this would upset her stomach. On occasions we would find items in the fridge that didn't belong there. Andrew had found a £20 note in the fridge which was a nice surprise. Other strange things happened in the kitchen such as finding empty yogurt cartons in the dish washer. Andrew's phone went missing and we were looking for hours, we phoned it and could hear a distant ring tone, we followed the muffled sound and eventually found it tucked away under the sink. We tolerated these events and found them mildly amusing. It certainly stopped us from leaving our phones on the worktops in the kitchen. Something had to be done though. One day I was returning from being outside and as I walked past the kitchen window I looked in and I could see Mum with a packet of ham in her hands, she was eating the handfuls of ham directly from the packet. This gorging was only one hour after she had eaten her breakfast and was totally unnecessary. So I tapped on the window gently to let her know that I was there. She looked up in panic, then she stuffed the ham that she was grasping back into its packet and quickly put it back in the fridge. She knew she was not supposed to be gorging on ham and so she was trying to hide the evidence quickly. I came through the door and questioned her;

'What have you just been eating?'

'Nowt.'

'You have, I have just seen you push the ham back into its packet.'

'Who are you telling me what to do, cossin me like a kid?'

' It's not nice Mum, you handling the ham and putting it back in the fridge.'

'Stop ,mithering, it's just a bit of snappin.'

'That's enough Mum, stop.'

Mum's Mow Cop, Staffordshire dialect became really strong when she was angry or when she had been caught out. Nowt is a Stoke word meaning nothing. Cossin means telling someone off. Mithering means fussing or nagging and Snappin means food. We had noticed that Mum had started to become agitated and aggressive in her tone of voice especially if things weren't going her way or if she had been found to be doing something she shouldn't.

The ham incident was the last straw for us with regard to fridge raiding as it was making us both feel quite nauseated. We were also very concerned that although she always washed her hands after going to the toilet, she was sometimes forgetful and had to be prompted to do so. The last thing we wanted was food poisoning and the thought of eating ham that had been in someone's fist was just too much. We also had to consider Mum's health, gorging on food is just not healthy and could lead to her having an upset stomach as well as excessive weight gain which would affect her already limited mobility. We decided that we needed to lock the fridge. Andrew ordered a child safe fridge lock and fitted it. He stood back and looked very proud of his work. As soon as we went out of sight, Mum tried to get into the fridge and found it to be locked. She was fuming and used that much force that whilst we were out of sight she yanked and pulled at the door until the child lock broke. She literally had ripped the lock off and it hung there all limp. When we came back into the kitchen she was very proud of the breakage.

'Huh, there, what are you going to do about that then?' she said laughing. She was so angry with us but we tried to explain that she could eat what she wanted and she only had to ask but we needed to lock the fridge to stop her gorging. She complained bitterly that we were treating her like a baby. Andrew was determined to put an end to the fridge raiding and this now became a battle of minds. So he purchased a more robust lock which she couldn't break. This was slightly annoying for us because we had to keep using a combination of numbers to undo the lock every time we wanted anything out of the fridge. We used to leave Mum some milk in a jug next to the kettle so she could always make herself a drink of tea though. We told her a white lie that we had to lock the fridge to stop someone from stealing food out of the fridge.

'Well I bet it is one of your boys or one of those girls.' By this she meant the carers. After that she seemed to accept that the fridge was now locked.

After the first Covid pandemic Lockdown, during August 2020, the government devised an incentive to help pubs and restaurants survive the loss of business they had suffered through enforced closure in the early phase of the pandemic. This incentive was called 'Eat Out to Help Out'. The idea was to help hospitality to re-open following the first Lockdown and was designed to boost this industry and to help secure hospitality jobs. Allister owns half a gastro pub business, The Barbridge Inn which is on the Chester Road 5 miles outside of Nantwich. Allister decided to take Mum out to his pub for lunch which would be enjoyable for Mum and it would also help the pub. The Barbridge is in a beautiful rural setting on the Shropshire Union canal and there are often traditional barges moored up outside. Mum and Dad used to love going to the pub for their lunch and the staff were always lovely with them. So on this particular day, Allister came over and took Mum in the car to the pub for a few hours. This was a welcome break for Andrew and me, and it meant that I could go out with my horse and do what I love which is compete in a dressage competition without worrying about Mum. Outdoor competitions were now allowed during this period of the pandemic. This was opened up after the initial strict rule of only being allowed to exercise for one hour per day. It felt so good to be able to get out and about again, it was invigorating. I felt like a captured bird who was now set free to fly.

After a few hours Allister returned Mum and he told us how she had really enjoyed her roast dinner as well as a change of scenery. It had been a successful mission and so off he went in his car to go home. He hadn't seen a lot of Mum early on in the pandemic as he was not allowed to travel over to our house which was about 8 miles away. Mum told me she had had a lovely afternoon and she seemed very content. When I took Mum to get washed and ready for bed I picked up her handbag which seemed rather heavy. Mum always carried her handbag around with her and had a caddy to put it in on her Zimmer frame.

'What's in here Mum?'

'Nowt.'

'It's very heavy, what's inside?'

I opened up the handbag to discover the whole of her roast dinner wrapped in serviettes, rolled up and hidden in her bag. Slightly leaking gravy.

'Why have you put your dinner in your handbag, Mum?'

' I anna put anything in the handbag.'

'Well, you must have done so because no one else would have.'

'I don't know who put it in there but it wanna me.'

Now I knew she was guilty because the Mow Cop dialect was coming out strong again. 'Anna' means I have not and 'wanna me' means it was not me. I know that when Allister goes to his pub he always visits the kitchen to see the chef and his co-owner James. I surmised that what probably happened is that Mum was either over faced by the amount of food or she wasn't enjoying her dinner. Mum was brought up with the principles that leaving food on her plate was not only wasteful but it was also rude. So she must have waited until Allister was not in view and quickly wrapped up the food and stuffed it in her handbag. On Allister's return from the kitchen she had smacked her lips and had told him how much she had enjoyed the food. The serviettes were sodden with gravy which had leaked into her bag. I cleaned the handbag as best I could and gave Bowie the roast dinner. Allister's adventure out to the pub wasn't quite as successful as he had believed. Bowie was very happy with the result though.

After the pub incident I became wise to the handbag trick and I used to have to watch out for her hoarding food in handbag. I would tell her to leave what she didn't want on the plate but I knew I was wasting my breath as the reinforced belief that you had to eat everything on her plate ran deep. If the handbag was not an option, she had another cunning plan. When Mum thought I wasn't looking she would do a perfect back handed flick of whatever food was on her fork in the direction of Bowie.

'Don't throw Bowie food Mum, it might upset his stomach.'

'I anna.'

'Yes, you have, I have just seen you.'

'He must have found sommat on the floor.'

'I saw you do it and it's not nice to do that at the dining table.'

'You are always cossin me, I canna do anything right.'

There was that Mow Cop tongue again, 'sommat' means something. This strong dialect was a sure sign that she knew what she was doing was wrong but she didn't want to leave the food on her plate. Bowie in the meantime looked pleased with himself and licked his lips. He didn't mind the flicking of food. I have to say, she was very good at it though, very precise. I would spy her out of the corner of my eye, looking to see if I was watching, if I was, the food would stay but if she thought I wasn't watching she would flick. I had to smile at her cunning and relentless pursuit to hide or get rid of her food. Seriously though, I was concerned that she may give Bowie something that may be poisonous to dogs and so I had to be vigilant at mealtimes.

On another occasion following a shopping trip to the supermarket, we were in the kitchen at home and I noticed a rectangle shape in Mum's cardigan sleeve.

'What is that up your sleeve, Mum?'

'Nowt.'

' There is definitely something up your sleeve.'

Mum's baby pink woollen cardigan had a definite rectangle shape of approximately 30cm x 12cm x 12cm going from the sleeve cuff to past her elbow on her left arm. It was acting like a splint and she couldn't bend her elbow.

'Come here and let me look at what's up your sleeve.'

'There's nowt to look at.'

On closer examination the rectangle was solid and the cardigan was straining and tight. I put my fingers inside the sleeve to feel cardboard and proceeded to pull the cardboard out. I delivered a slightly squashed Morrison's lemon cake out of that sleeve. I don't know who was more shocked, me or Mum.

'Well, how did that get up there?'

'I don't know Mum, you tell me.'

'Well, fancy that being up there.'

The cake just didn't have the same appeal as it was flattened under the strain of the cardigan. Unfortunately, the cake had to be thrown away because it was so squashed and inedible. Lots of food items went into Mum's handbag, coat pockets or up her sleeve. Food hoarding and stealing became a leisure pursuit for Mum. I would frequently find food items in Mum's pockets. I could not understand why she was trying to throw food away or hide it one minute and at other times she was stealing food.

Sharon used to take Mum out in her car for a drive to prevent boredom for both of them, to act as a distraction for Mum and to perform errands. Mum loved a drive out in the car, she would take in the scenery and be quiet and content. Sharon was also a horsey person and I had met her via our connections with other horse friends. Sharon would take Mum with her to run her errands or she would take her to watch the dressage at one of the local equestrian centres called Beaver Hall. Beaver Hall Equestrian centre is situated outside Leek at Bradnop on the way to Ashbourne. It is often cold up there, it can be windy and frequently rains but there is always a warm welcome inside the café. Sharon used to sit Mum outside and wrap her in a horse blanket to keep her warm or Mum would wait in the car if it was cold, windy or raining and on occasions they would sit in the cafe. Sharon and Mum became an infamous pair locally. The only problem with Sharon leaving Mum in her car was that it left Mum alone and she was able to get up to mischief. Sharon stored some snacks and sweets in the glove compartment of her car. Quite often Sharon would telephone me in the evening to ask me to check Mum's coat pockets for a chocolate bar that she had been looking forward to eating later after work. I would go and check Mum's coat pockets and there it would be. Mum always claimed to know nothing about how it got there. Mum used to eat her way through a bag of sweets that were Sharon's without a second thought. One day, Sharon and Mum had returned to the house after collecting the horse feed for Sharon's horse, Maisey. Mum was desperate for the toilet so Sharon took her to the bathroom in order to avoid an accident. When Sharon helped Mum to pull down her pants, hundreds of 5 pences started to fall out of her clothing like a slot machine in an amusement arcade.

'What's happening here, Sybil?'

'I dunna know.'

'Where is all this money coming from?'

Sharon realised then that this money belonged to her and that Mum had taken the bag of 5 pences that she kept in the glove compartment of the car. When I got home, Sharon told me about Mum literally spending pennies when she went to the toilet. We did laugh but this stealing was getting out of hand. That evening after Sharon had gone home, I took Mum for a shower. When I helped her undress more 5 pences came out of her clothing, out of her bra and jumper and they rolled along the floor. We were finding 5 pences for months after that.

Chapter 12

The Conservatory

When we had moved into the house we had always intended to renew the conservatory because of its leaking roof. It leaked so badly that water used to pour down the walls, we had buckets and towels on the floor situated in various spots around the conservatory ready to catch the water. However, we couldn't afford to renew it because there were so many other things that needed doing first and were a higher priority. The renewal of the conservatory was on page 4 of our long term project list. However, when Mum came to live with us it became more of a priority as that is where Mum liked to sit and where she would spend most of her day. It was also where the dining table was and where Mum ate her meals. In the Staffordshire Moorlands it frequently rains and sometimes the rain is torrential. One day, Mum was in the conservatory eating some homemade leek and potato soup. Homemade soup was Mum's favourite meal and nothing would stop Mum from eating. All of a sudden the heavens opened and the rain was pouring down, the conservatory couldn't cope with the amount of water so it began to leak badly. Water was pouring down the walls and it was also coming through the joints in the conservatory roof just above where Mum was sitting. We had buckets placed around the conservatory to catch the water and whilst Mum finished her soup, Andrew stood with a bucket above her head. She seemed oblivious to what was going on around her.

I felt terrible that Mum was expected to live in a house where her main living room had a leaking roof and it was damp. We decided that we had to renew the conservatory and soon. The obvious answer was to use some of the money from Mum's house sale to build Mum a comfortable and warm oak room and Allister agreed to this. It was essential that Mum was comfortable and that she was kept as safe as possible. We had become Mum's carers and our home was her home now.

'You deserve to have a nice oak room for looking after Mum,' Allister said.

I contacted the builders and after a month or so, they tore down the old conservatory which was made of PVC and glass. As a temporary measure, we moved the dining table and chairs into the hall which was a bit of a squeeze but hopefully this would not be for long. The builders told us that the erecting an oak room was quite a quick project. Unfortunately, the foundation stage of building did not go to plan and took much longer than anticipated. The builder kept digging down, deeper and deeper but they could not find a solid platform to build on. The surveyors came and puzzled over this until they decided that we needed a floating platform which would hold the weight of the oak. This was both costly and took a long time to complete. Mum loved having extra people around though. The builders were fair game for Mum as she liked to talk to people. If Mum was left alone whilst I nipped out to see to the horses, Mum would open the door and shout to the builders,

'Help, Help!'

'Hello. What's the matter?'

'I'm lost and I'm looking for Alan, have you seen him?'

The builders would come to find me and say that Mum was distressed and shouting 'Help'.

'Don't worry, she is alright.'

'Who's Alan?'

'That was my Dad, you will just have to ignore her and I will be back in the house in a few minutes.'

These regular interruptions did not do anything to speed up the build. The builders would try to carry on with their work but they were too polite to ignore Mum and so she had a captive audience. One of the builders was young, very polite and very patient with Mum. She would ask them if they wanted a drink, ask them where they lived and whether they knew Alsager or Mow Cop. She constantly distracted them from what they were doing. She would constantly ask them if they had seen me or her husband, Alan.

Mum also acted like a supervisor, foreman or auditor and could be very critical of the builders' work. The electrician, Mick, was in the kitchen one evening looking at the circuit board, looking puzzled as he tried to work out what was wrong following a power cut. Mum, Andrew and myself were in the kitchen with candle lights and torches. The kitchen was also where the circuit board is and Mick was standing up a ladder, peering at the circuit.

'Calls himself an Electrician, look at him, he hasn't got a clue.'

'Shush Mum, don't be rude.'

Then a bit louder,

'I shan't shush, he hasn't a clue, he has no idea.'

I could see Mick chuckle. The builders were extremely patient and over the following few months they became quite fond of Mum. They looked out for her when they knew she was on her own despite her spiteful remarks about their work. Sharon would make the builders cups of tea in the day and there was plenty of laughter. Mum loved the attention and having people around her. The gradual building of the conservatory provided her with daily entertainment.

Eventually the foundation was complete and the floor was stable enough to take the weight of the oak and glass. This meant that a different team of people came who specialised in oak frames. The oak room was built by two very polite and capable young men, Charlie and Ben. These were fresh meat for Mum and new people meant additional entertainment and as soon as she was left alone for a short while she would engage with them.

'Hello (posh voice), do you think you could help me!'

'Hello. Are you alright?'

'No, they have left me all alone and I'm lost, where am I?'

'You are at home, you live with Isabel.'

Charlie and Ben were really concerned and came to find me at the stables and I explained that Mum quite often said this as she didn't like me going to the stables and leaving her alone even for a few minutes. If this didn't work she would try:

'Hello, boys, can you help me?'

'We can try.'

'Have you seen Alan? I don't know where he is. He is always doing this.'

The poor boys were totally out of their depth and had not had any involvement with someone with dementia. Mum would criticise them and their carpentry skills and say that Alan would have had this job finished by now.

'What are they messing about at?' She would say loudly so that they could hear.

Or she would completely throw them by asking,

'Where's my Blue Hat? I've lost it.'

It was on top of her head, she was wearing it but they were too polite to say. I would do my best to protect them from this barrage and let them get on with their work. The trouble was when I was at work I had no control and Sharon loved banter so she would encourage Mum. That summer of building the conservatory filled our house and garden with laughter. The weather was kind so Mum and Sharon could sit outside enjoying the sunshine. The Moorhens would race across the grass with their long legs, looking slightly ungainly and prehistoric. Rabbits would be munching on the grass and there were garden birds everywhere. Overhead you could see the buzzard and hear its long drawn out call 'Kee-aaah'. The insects would buzz and hover around the flowers and our small pond. The wildlife didn't seem to mind Mum, Sharon or the builders, everyone and everything was living in harmony. Mum loved the garden and when she was feeling up to it, she would do a bit of weeding the raised flower beds. The garden and surroundings at Lapwing Farm were idyllic so it was no wonder Mum felt content when she was living with us. She was also content when she had company especially when she had Sharon for company on the week days all to herself.

The oak beams for the new conservatory were soon erected once the foundations were sorted and so the finishing touches included large glass windows, a tiled floor and the roof tiles. The fireplace was re-opened and the room was decorated. The room also had bi-folding doors so that it could be kept cool in the summer months and under floor heating so that Mum would be warm in the winter. It was perfect and Mum loved it. This was Mum's special place. We placed Mum's rocking chair in the centre near to the window so she could watch the wildlife outside. We had birdfeeders placed just outside so that Mum could watch the Blue Tits, Finches and Chaffinches. They would dart from the prickly scrubs to the bird table and feeders for hours, there were so many of them it was impossible to count them. We had a wood pigeon as well that used to eat up all of the fallen seed. There were several cheeky squirrels that used to love stealing the nuts by hanging upside down from the top of the bird feeder. Bowie would go mad when he saw the squirrels and he would bounce on the back of the old leather sofas barking at them until he was banished from the room. Mum would just sit calmly observing what was going on in the garden as it was teaming with wildlife and she could spend hours doing this. Despite her Alzheimer's and her inability to remember names she retained the ability to identify certain birds. She would often tell me about what birds were in the garden. I would be fascinated as to what the brain decided to retain and what it lost.

On one occasion, I was in the kitchen and Mum was sitting comfortably in the conservatory when I heard a very fast knocking noise. I thought something had happened to Mum so I rushed in. No, nothing had happened to Mum, she was sitting contently. Then the rapid hollow tapping sound came again just outside. When I peered around the corner there was a beautiful Great Spotted Woodpecker hammering away on our new oak timber beams. He was beautiful with pied black and white plumage and a small red patch on the back on his head. I was thrilled that he liked our new conservatory but I couldn't let him continue to rapidly drum on the wood because I didn't want a hole making in the oak so I let him know I was there. The thing that I found most surprising about living in the countryside is that you feel like you are sharing the space of the wildlife and they are very relaxed about it. The ducks will argue and chase each other like you don't exist and now there was a Woodpecker close up, pecking away without any concern for being so close to the house. Once the Woodpecker had seen me, he flew off. I frequently hear him or other Woodpeckers in the surrounding trees. Mum didn't hear him at all even with her hearing aids in situ because she was quite hard of hearing particularly in the higher frequencies. Mum's hearing was damaged when she worked in the textile mill which was very noisy and there wasn't any hearing protection or health and safety law like there is now.

'Did you hear or see the Woodpecker, Mum?'

'No, I would have liked to have seen him.'

'He was beautiful, pecking away at the oak beam.'

Mum may have been able to retain some information about garden birds. However and unfortunately, Mum had started to lose people's names. She would frequently use the phrase 'whatsamajig' or 'whosamajig' when she was trying to remember a name and she would become cross with you for not knowing who she was talking about.

'You do know, whatsamajig, you know.'

'I don't know who you are talking about, sorry.'

'Oh! Never mind!'

I noticed that Mum had started a new phase of the Alzheimer's where she had started referring to me as someone else or talking about her daughter Isabel to me and calling me nurse. I used to have to remind her of who I was and where she was several times a day.

'Oh thank goodness you are here nurse, I'm lost.'

'You are not lost Mum, you are with me.'

'Yes but I am looking for Alan, have you seen him?'

That terrible pain hit me again out of the blue, the sudden grief of losing my beloved Dad.

'Alan's not here, do you remember what happened Mum?'

'Have you seen my daughter? She's a nurse too.'

'I am your daughter! Mum, I'm Isabel and Dad's not here anymore.'

'Oh yes, of course you are, I'm a silly bugger, Alan's dead isn't he?'

This sort of conversation would always be followed by silent reflection by both of us.

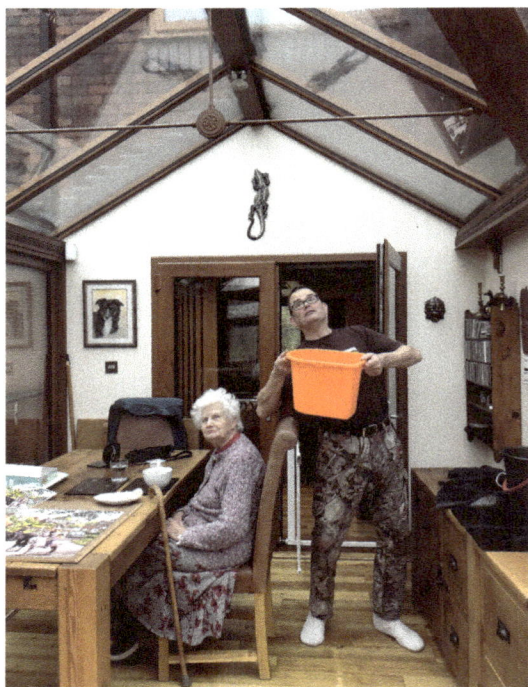

Andrew catching water in the leaking conservatory so that Mum could carry on eating

Chapter 13

Memories

Mum had moments when she was completely lucid which always caught me by surprise. Apparently this is called paradoxical lucidity and can happen even when a person has been unable to communicate for a while due to dementia. They will suddenly snap out of the locked up state of the brain that they have been experiencing. We know so little about how the brain really works, research is ongoing but a lot of findings are theory based rather than fact. During these moments of lucidity, Mum would be totally aware of her surroundings, of the people around her and she would be aware of her own strange behaviour. This would only last for a short while. She would say something like,

'You have been marvellous to me, you shouldn't have to put up with me'

At other times she would say,

'I was bloody crackers last night, behaving like that, why didn't you hit me over the head with a hammer?'

Inside that lost person was Mum who had a cracking sense of humour. I would then ask her a question but just as quickly as her clarity had come, it was gone again and we were back to confusion, agitation or worse, fear. As the Alzheimers progressed so did her anxiety and fear. Mum had never really been a tactile person but she started to want to sit and hold my hand. I would constantly reassure her that she was safe. I was her safety net though and when I had to leave her for a short while to go down to the stables to see to the horses she would follow with Bowie by her side on his lead. Mum wanted to be with me all of the time. Thank goodness for Bowie as he was a good substitute for me, he would sit with Mum and be tickled for hours. Bowie would stay with Mum and guard her in return for constant ear tickling. Some people with dementia like a blanket or piece of material to rub constantly, Mum had Bowies soft ears and he couldn't get enough of it.

Mum was better at remembering detail from her younger years but not so good at remembering more recent times or events. Her short term memory was non-existent. However, she loved to talk about years gone by and it used to light her up. Mum's first job when she was sixteen years old was working in a textile mill. The mill was called Conlowe's and it was situated next to the River Dane, in Congleton, Cheshire. Conlowe's was a very busy and noisy textile mill which was full of bobbins and cotton. It was based in an old mill called Dane Mill which was originally a corn mill dating back to the 19th century. In its day the mill had a waterwheel and a feeder canal from the River Dane, the waterwheel has long gone but the feeder canal is still there. The mill has been many things over the years but now it is full of small businesses. As a coincidence, one of the businesses is ours. So when we were going to work during the early Covid days and Mum was left in the house, she would constantly and repetitively ask questions about where we were going.

'We are going to work Mum, my telephone number is on the kitchen top, phone me if you need me'.

'Where are you going?'

'We are going to work and I have written down where we are going, the telephone number is written on the piece of paper and that we will be back at 5pm, we are working in Congleton at our business'.

'Where are you going?'

After about another five or six attempts to explain where we were going and what we were doing in our business, I gave up.

'We are going to work, in Conlowe's'

'Oh, that's good, I used to work in Conlowe's, see you later!'

This would satisfy Mum and she would be content with the answer and then she would settle. In the evening we would talk about Conlowe's and the time that she worked there. She had a photograph of when she worked in the mill with all of her friends. We could recognise the structure of the building, the interior had changed and made into smaller offices but the building was much the same. When Ash came up from London during the first Covid Lockdown to get away from the London crowds, he would come into work with Andrew and I. Ashley didn't like to tell Mum lies and say that we were going to Conlowe's so he tried to tell her where we were going.

'Where are you going, are you going as well Ashley?'

'Yes, we are going to work in Congleton at Dane Mill'

'Where are you going?'

He tried to explain and was very patient but in the end he also realised and came around to saying;

'We are going Conlowe's to work'

'I used to work there, I bet it has changed over the years, it's been going for some years that place has, fancy you working there too'

In the evenings I would sit with Mum and try to help her with her recall. Memories are extremely precious and I wanted to try to preserve any memories that she had. Some days were better than others. I had taken all the photographs and documents from Mum and Dad's house when she had moved into our home with us. So I got an old wooden box and created a memory box. Mum had saved everything, there were newspaper clips from World War 2, ration books, Dad's National Service record but there were also other people's death certificates. I had no idea who some of these people were and Mum couldn't enlighten me either. We would spend hours going through the box. I was fascinated with this historical collection of documents and got as much enjoyment out of going through the box as Mum did. I would watch Mum's face light up as she remembered and told me stories of the past. There were photographs of when she was at school and in a pantomime and she could remember all about it and pointed out a few other people in the photo. The memory box helped Mum to recall people and events and it was lovely to see her eyes brighten and her brain relight. I had also saved some old tins out of her pantry in Alsager which must have been fifty plus years old. They looked like they should have been in a museum. I would bring these out and we would discuss what they were used for and she would reminisce. I also bought a few Cd's with old fashioned songs on. I would play these and Mum would sing along, remembering all of the words. It's strange how music can bring people with dementia out of the world that they are locked in. Mum's face would light up as she remembered what the songs meant to her. She would even do some of the actions associated with certain songs such as waving her hands during a song called "when you are smiling" or pretending to blow bubbles to the "I'm forever blowing bubbles" song.

During the Covid pandemic time it was very hard for Mum to be present. This period of time was very disconcerting and isolating for everyone but for a person suffering from Alzheimers the isolation was dreadful and very damaging. Trying to help a person to make sense of their surroundings and of their community became near enough impossible. We all became very insular which compounded the symptoms of confusion and withdrawal. Mum's friend Thelma used to telephone but Mum was losing the ability to understand who someone was unless she could see them. I had started to notice that she was struggling to recognise people. Sometimes she referred to me as Thelma. As we came out of Lockdown we were able to visit familiar places in the car. I drove Mum over to Alsager and we parked up outside of her old house to talk to her old neighbours. Mum seemed to enjoy doing this but I was unsure whether she actually recognised who the neighbours were or whether she was just bluffing. It's embarrassing for anyone when you can't remember someone you meet especially when they are not in context and I'm sure this happens to us all from time to time but for a person with Alzheimers this is reality, however, Mum still had the feeling of 'I should know this person' and therefore, I will pretend I know who they are. When we parked outside her old house, it didn't spark any emotions, I thought she may be sad because the new owners hadn't cared for her beloved garden but there wasn't any reaction. We also went to visit a few of her friends who lived in Alsager. We went to see Thelma and Anthony at their house, we sat in the garden for a cup of tea and a piece of cake. This was during the time that you were allowed to visit in an outside space whilst keeping a 2 metre distance away from each other. Mum loved her visit and she seemed to remember the stories that went back to her Caretaker days in the school.

We would call in at Aunty Pam's house every week to take her the weekly shop and to have a chat. Mum and Aunty Pam were cousins and they had known each other all of their lives. Aunty Pam didn't see the dementia so they just chatted away for an hour. I took Mum to visit her brother, George who was a few years older than her. Uncle George and Mum hadn't seen each other for months because of the pandemic. He still lived in the same village that they had grown up in, Mow Cop. George's health was deteriorating as well, he had lost one of his legs following a hospital blunder a few years back but he still managed to live on his own independently. He couldn't really get out and about because the roads were steep in the village but he managed to wheel himself around his bungalow. Aunty Dorothy, his wife, had died a few years previously. She was the love of his life and her death had hit him hard but he was strong and he had soldiered on without her. Mum recognised George and it was as if they had never been parted. They both really enjoyed these rare visits and you could see how close they were. During these visits the Alzheimers was less obvious and the companionship did Mum the world of good. These visits used a lot of Mum's energy so when we returned home she would go and sit in the conservatory contented for a few hours and she would have a nap.

During the summer months and when the weather was kind we spent a lot of time outside. Sometimes, some of Allister's children would visit with their children. Mum loved children, she would love seeing them but I'm not convinced that she knew who they were. Mum loved being outside when the weather was good. She would sit on the patio and watch the wildlife but Mum's favourite place was either sitting next to our small pond or sitting outside the stables. At the stables, we would watch the comical Oyster Catchers, there were three of them and they used to sit on a fence post each or they would chase each other around. They make a very distinctive peep, peep, peep noise and they always made us laugh. They didn't really care about our presence either, I don't think they saw us as a threat. On the odd occasion we also had Lapwings come to visit but they tended to stay on the large Mill Pond next door. The stables are full of Swallow nests in the summer and they swoop around, again they don't care about us being around. They would swoop in and out of the stables showing a fantastic aerodynamic display. Their chicks would be waiting for a feed and four or five beaks would hang out of the nests waiting for their parents. On the large pond there are a mixture of Mallard ducks, Tufted ducks, Moorhens, Coots and Canadian Geese. What is living in or around the pond depends on the time of year and there seems to be the same cycle which we hadn't yet worked out. There was a lot of rabbits in the garden who used to run off when Bowie was outside but I don't think they were that bothered by him, he loved the chase and that was all. We even found a Newt living under some wood. Later in the year we have thousands of toadlets that leave our pond, they head across the garden and make their way down to the stream at the bottom of the garden. Insects of all descriptions are abundant all around us. All these wildlife cycles were happening in our garden and on our land, it was incredible to witness.

So when the weather was good I would get the folding chairs out so that me and Mum could sit and just live in the moment enjoying the peace of the countryside whilst observing the wildlife which was all around us. I would get us both a cup of tea. We were lucky to live in such a beautiful setting with such freedom during the Lockdowns. I couldn't help but to feel very fortunate. Some people were stuck in high rise flats and that must have been so difficult in Lockdown. Sitting with Mum was quality time and it reminded me of the quality time that I was fortunate to experience with Dad. Sitting outside near to the stables listening to the horses snorting softly was perfect. It was also a good opportunity to get some jobs done so we would spend time cleaning horse tack, buckets or grooming brushes. This was very useful as well as a pleasant way to spend time with Mum. During the good weather we used to garden together. Andrew had cut an old sherry barrel in half and made a couple of large planters. Mum really enjoyed planting the bedding plants and weeding the pots. These are the special times that I will always remember. The only problem was that usually these occasions lasted about an hour and then:

'We had better go back, Alan will wonder where I am, sitting here doing nowt'

'Mum, Dad is not waiting for you, don't you remember what happened to Dad'

'Well we better get back and start his tea'

People in the north often refer to their evening meal as tea rather than dinner. This comes from the olden days where people had low tea or high tea. Afternoon tea or low tea became a thing in Victorian times when the ladies of the household became peckish in the afternoon but they didn't want a large meal. This became popular in high society which eventually filtered down to the working class. Whereas high tea was really dinner and involved a snack and a main meal. After a period of time it became common for the working class to call their midday meal 'dinner' and their evening meal 'tea'. The upper class called their midday meal 'lunch' and their evening meal 'dinner'. These days some people use a mixture of both and this is no longer dependant on class. In our family, we were definitely dinner and tea, we never lunched.

⚫

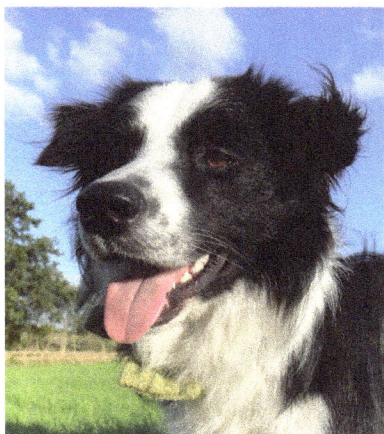

Bowie

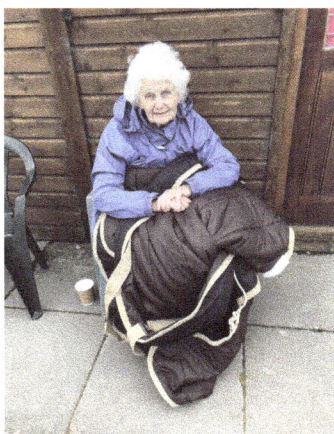

Mum watching
dressage at Beaver Hall
Equestrian Centre

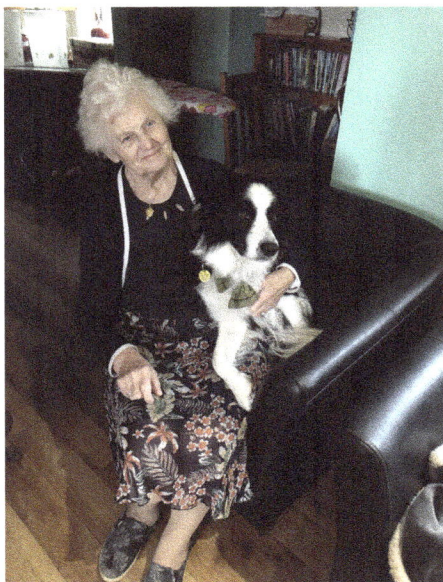

Mum and Bowie

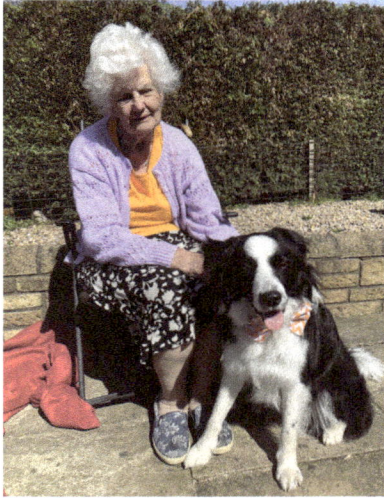

Bowie and Mum enjoying the sunshine

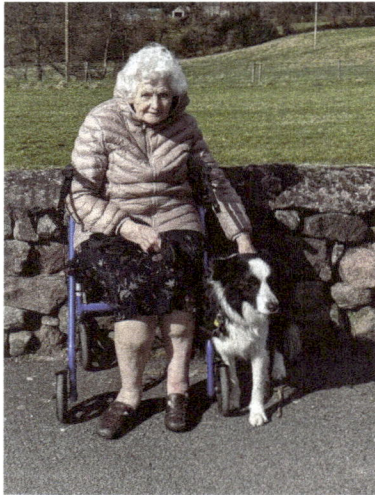

Mum taking Bowie for a short walk

Chapter 14

Doppelgangers

As Mum's dementia progressed,Andrew and I became at least two or three people. Andrew had become three other people depending on what day it was. Mum would recognise Andrew as my husband, who was a respectable person and who was a good son-in-law. On rare occasions, and very worryingly for Andrew, Mum would refer to him as her own husband. It was a good job that Mum wasn't tactile, otherwise I think Andrew would have freaked out. However, his other doppelgangers had less favourable reviews from Mum. Andrew became the gardener with little or no idea of what he was doing and she would use her favourite spiteful saying;

'Call himself a Gardener, huh, he has no idea!'.

'There is no need to be like that, it's unkind. Don't be nasty Mum'

'Well, look at him, doesn't know a flower from a weed, hopeless!'

Andrew was also the man who came to do DIY. Andrew doesn't like DIY at the best of times but when you have a bit of land you have to do quite a lot of it. The horses can be very destructive as well and there are always fences to repair and fence posts to knock in. Mum was very critical of his DIY capabilities, she didn't help him to like it, she didn't encourage him and would be just down right rude.

She would snigger and say 'look at him, useless! I have seen more work in a Becham's Pill'

Andrew and I were very confused by this strange saying but if you look it up on google, it is there under strange Stoke-on-Trent dialect, it means that the person is lazy. Andrew is not lazy and he is always doing jobs around the place when he isn't working in his normal work role. You could not stop her from saying these spiteful comments though and she seemed to really enjoy herself when she was being highly critical. I would try to talk to her and say that it wasn't nice but that just made her worse and she would justify her reasoning by pointing out what he was doing wrong. I couldn't work out if this was my Mum's true feelings being expressed or whether this was part of the dementia. She had become a professional auditor with no filter. Mum used this saying a lot about the builders when they were erecting the oak conservatory, not so much about the boys because she really liked them but definitely about their boss. Their boss used to turn up late in the morning approximately 2 hours after the boys had been working. He would order Charlie and Ben about but would never actually do any of the work himself. Mum latched on to this and would be lovely about the two young men but she was not very complementary about their boss. She would make comments about him and the boys would chuckle and this just encouraged her to say more less complementary things about him. She seemed to love being critical and in the spotlight.

'No work in him'. This was her favourite saying when auditing people's work.

'His mouth works though, no problem there, lots of gas'.

This last comment had Charlie and Ben in bulk with laughter.

Andrew's last doppelganger was the guitar player. Andrew was learning to play the guitar and thought that during Lockdown, it would be an excellent time to learn. This was not so easy with Mum sitting nearby and commenting. I was also learning to play the piano and I had been doing this on and off for a number of years. When Cameron was little my Dad had bought me a piano and I had taken a few grades. I can read music but I have never really got to grips with playing the piano and I don't have a natural ear for music, I rely on reading music scripts. I would play a tune on the piano and Mum would sit there listening to me and make positive remarks. The music I played was much slower than it should be and if I'm honest I really wasn't very good. I had a fear of playing the piano in front of strangers but I enjoyed it and it felt therapeutic for me which is what counts. When you are reading music and playing the piano, you can't think of anything else and it makes you very present. Mum was my only audience and she would tap her foot as I played.

'That's lovely, play it again'

'Ok, just for you'.

However, when Mum was listening to Andrew play the guitar, she kept putting him off.

'No tune in him, ha-ha'

'Mum, don't be so rude'

'He will have the cats out calling if he carries on, no tune in him'.

Andrew's enthusiasm for learning the guitar soon dwindled, not particularly because of Mum but it must have been off putting. I used to tease him as I received the compliments she gave to me and I had to laugh about what she said about Andrew's guitar playing.

Now I know, I am not a good piano player and I never play in front of other people but you have to take the compliments where you can. I would look at Andrew with a smug look on my face when I received the compliments. Mum loved Andrew though in any form that he was taking on any given day and the hassle that she gave him was only in jest.

I had also become three people. I was me, the loving daughter, the one that she couldn't do without. Mum would cling to me and fret whenever I had to go anywhere without her. I was also the matron of the nursing home that she believed she was living in. Mum and Dad had always called me matron as a joke. As I approached, Dad used to say,

'Stand by your beds! Matron is here'

I don't know if this is where Mum got the idea of me being the matron of the nursing home she was living in. Mum would call to me in her very polite and best posh voice.

'Excuse me, Sister, please could you help me, I'm' lost'

'You are not lost Mum, you are with me, I'm your daughter, remember'.

'That's good, of course you are. I don't know how you are making enough money here though, I'm the only person in here'

'In where Mum'

'Well you and Andrew have set up this nursing home and I'm worried that it isn't doing very well'

'Well Mum, we are in Lockdown and no one else is allowed here'

'Is that right, well I don't know how you are going to make any money. Where's Alan, is he not allowed to be here either?'

'No Mum, don't you remember…'.

Again, the pain of grief would hit me and I would have to feel the reoccurring emotions of losing Dad.

Sometimes, I was The Carer who was not a very good carer. I would be trying to get Mum to do something that she didn't want to do. Whatever it was that I was asking her to do was not being received well.

'I am going to report you'

'oh really and who are you going to report me to? I am trying to help you'.

'I am going to report you to Isabel Burrows'

At this point I would have to laugh.

'Mum, I am Isabel Burrows, your daughter'.

'Don't be so ridiculous, what a ridiculous thing to say, just wait until she gets here, she is in charge of this place you know, she will sort you out, she is the Matron'.

As the Alzheimer's dementia progressed these outbursts became more frequent. Sharon was not a trained carer, she did her best but she did struggle with these outbursts. Sometimes they would end up arguing and Sharon would telephone me because Mum had upset her. I gave Sharon a computer and enrolled her on a care course so that she would understand Mum's needs better. I was also aware that this was a one way ticket for Mum and once she was gone, so was Sharon's work. So, I thought a qualification would provide Sharon with better prospects that she could use after Mum had gone. By 'Gone', I mean when and after Mum had died.

Mum was becoming increasingly awkward, this happened more at night but it was also starting to happen more in the daytime as well. Quite often I would be at work trying to help our customers navigate through the Covid pandemic and I would receive a phone call from Sharon. Sharon would tell me that Mum was being difficult and argumentative and I would try to calm the situation down by reassuring Sharon that it was not personal but part of the dementia.

'Hi, Sharon, are you OK?'

'I can't do this anymore'

'Why, what's the matter?'

'Your Mum hates me and she has told me that I'm useless and she is going to report me to Isabel Burrows'

'Sharon, Mum doesn't even know who I am anymore, she doesn't hate you, it's just the dementia, she doesn't really know who you are'

'But if she tells you things that I have done, when I haven't, you are going to think bad of me'

'Don't worry, I know it's not true and anyway she reports me to you. And she is going to report me to Isabel Burrows as well. It's just part of the dementia, please don't worry'

'OK, I hope you don't mind me phoning you at work?'

'No, not at all. I don't know who this Isabel Burrows is but she seems very strict, Ha Ha'.

This reassurance usually worked well and when I returned home instead of a war I would find peace and harmony as they tried to find a jigsaw piece together. Sometimes after Sharon had gone home Mum would talk about her day with Sharon.

'Between you and me, she is bloody crackers, she thinks I'm crackers, well she needs to look at herself'

'What do you mean?'

'She is funny, she makes me laugh but she is bloody crackers'.

Mum would say someone is 'Bloody Crackers' in an affectionate way and it was strangely a compliment. It was times like this when Mum seemed to be her old self and quite lucid. Mum got on well with Sharon and Mum loved their trips out as well as her company. In the day, Mum was fairly settled despite the odd outburst.

The evenings, however, were becoming more difficult. Mum was constantly trying to get more food to gorge on, trying to find Dad and saying that she didn't feel very well. Meal times were difficult mainly because we liked different types of food including spicey food, whereas, Mum liked simple traditional food. Mum also expected to eat at the same time each day and couldn't cope with eating at 7pm as she thought that was too late. I would end up cooking different meals and at different times to accommodate this. When we got home I would attempt to relax and unwind after a full day at work but I would constantly have to keep getting up to go to see to Mum. She would tell me that she felt unwell but she couldn't describe what was wrong. It was difficult to decide whether she was actually unwell or trying to attract attention. I tried to ask her questions of how she felt and what she meant by feeling unwell.

'I just feel No How',

'What do you mean by No How?'

'You know, So, So'

'I don't know what So, So means, Mum, try to explain. Do you have any pain?'

'I don't know, I can't explain but I don't feel well'

I would go to have a relaxing bath and then I would hear the jingle which meant that Mum was in the kitchen raiding.

Man it doesn't show signs of stopping

And I brought me some corn for popping

The lights are turned way down low

Let it snow! Let it snow! Let it snow!

Then I could hear crashing coming from the kitchen. I would jump out of the bath, with a dripping wet body and hair, throw a towel around me and rush down the stairs to find out what the crash was and what Mum was doing. I would ask Mum to go back to her bedroom as she had only just had her tea and could not be hungry. On other occasions as soon as I had lowered myself in to the bath, she would shout,

'Help me, HELP' in a very dramatic manner to make me believe that she had fallen. I tried to ignore her thinking that this is what she does when she is left alone but it was impossible. I would have to go to see if she was alright. I would jump out of the bath dripping wet, pull a towel around me, water dripping and my feet were making the carpet wet. I would run down the stairs to find her safe.

'What is wrong, I thought you had fallen'

'I'm Lost, I'm in trouble and I don't know where I am, can you help me, Nurse'

I could feel myself becoming annoyed and had to take a deep breath. I had to think of a distraction.

'Mum, you are safe just go and sit down, I will be downstairs in a few minutes. Funny Man's on tonight and we can watch it together'

'Oh good I like him'

I would go back upstairs to finish my bath and sort myself out, giving up on my relaxing bath time. When I came back downstairs, we would all go into the front room and I would let Mum have the best seat whilst we watched TV together. I would put Michael McIntyre's Big Show on. Mum was unable to follow stories, films or any complex quiz's but she loved the Big Show. She would laugh out loud and call him 'The Funny Man'. So we used to watch this every Saturday night when it was on. I would get Mum, her favourite alcoholic drink which was a glass of Croft Original sherry. No other sherry would do, it had to be Croft Original. I would have one too and as I drank it, it warmed my inner core and gave me the feeling of safety and comfort. Mum had a glass of sherry every night and it became a ritual, she had a glass every night without fail. I would then help Mum to get ready for bed and tuck her up in her favourite chair, the bed next to her empty as she still refused to sleep in it. As a qualified nurse I worried that she might develop pressure sores from the prolonged sitting all day and night but I just couldn't persuade her to sleep in the bed. She would tell me that she would sleep in the bed tomorrow night. She would tell me this every night but she did seem happy and comfortable. I would sit with Mum until she started to doze off and then I would sneak out to go to watch television with Andrew. However, as soon as I sat down, she would wake up and be on the move again. It was exhausting.

⌖

Chapter 15

Respite

During the Covid lockdown I remember seeing an elderly man on the BBC news who was living with his wife who had Alzheimer's. He was at breaking point and I remember feeling empathy for him. I felt like I wanted to help him and I would have done if I could have. He was in a desperate state, I felt so sorry for him but it wasn't sympathy that he wanted, it was help that he needed. Help was not available though. You could tell that he truly loved his wife, he didn't want to give up on her by putting her in a nursing home. He wanted to care for her himself and he wanted her to stay in her own home which was familiar to her. I could identify with him as I was also really worried about Mum going into a nursing home due to the risk of contracting Covid. However, I was exhausted and I needed a break! I just needed to work out how we could arrange this and when was the best time whilst keeping Mum safe. On the news every night during the early days of the Covid pandemic there were figures released of the number of Covid deaths for that day. The numbers were high. It was terrifying and it changed the way people viewed and behaved towards other people. The only places where you really made contact with other people was in the supermarket at that time. If someone came too close to you or leaned across you to reach something on a shelf, you would quickly jump away. Everyone was suspicious of other people particularly if they coughed. I have mild asthma and sometimes I would be trying to stifle a cough. The more you tried not to cough, the more you wanted to cough, it became psychosomatic.

The hospitals were in crisis and needed to admit people to the Intensive Care Units (ICU). All over the country, the hospital beds were full and there was a major shortage of ICU beds. I had never experienced anything like this before during the whole of my nursing career. Staffing was desperately short due to staff testing positive to Covid or through exhaustion. During this crisis and mainly because of the shortage of beds, the powers to be, came up with a plan which was to utilise nursing homes. The nursing homes had some capacity to take more people but what they didn't have was sufficient training in dealing with infection control and barrier nursing through isolation. The majority of the staff in nursing homes are non-qualified care assistants who have some basic awareness of pathogens and basic infection control through hand washing and PPE. These care assistants do an amazing job caring for people but this crisis was off the scale and the infection control requirements and skills required were extreme compared to anything they had done previously. During the early stages of the pandemic, the nursing homes and the hospitals were vastly short of appropriate and sufficient Personal Protection Equipment (PPE) such as aprons, hand sanitiser, gloves or Respiratory Protective Equipment (RPE) called FFP3 masks. The nursing homes certainly didn't have Face Fit testing to test if the masks were actually working and they had very little time to provide adequate training for unqualified staff of donning and doffing PPE and RPE. Donning is a term used for putting on PPE whilst being careful not to contaminate it and doffing means removing it whilst being extremely careful not to contaminate and cause cross infection. Covid-19 is an airborne virus and it is spread through air droplets when someone sneezes or coughs as well as through touch with contaminated hands. I am not being critical of the government, the policy makers or the carers as these were unprecedented times but the result of releasing Covid patients into nursing homes was catastrophic. In a report produced by the Office of National Statistics, it was reported that deaths involving Covid-19 in the care sector for England and Wales between the week ending 20 March 2020 and week ending 21 January 2022 were 45,632 which equated to 16.7% of deaths in the care homes. There was a direct correlation between elderly people with Covid-19 being moved from hospitals into the nursing homes and with the increase of deaths in the nursing homes by 30% in the first and second wave of the pandemic. The death statistics were being calculated and announced on the television on the evening BBC news at 10pm every night and it was terrifying. People were dying in hospitals or in nursing homes without their family being with them at their bedside and sometimes they died when they were totally alone. In the early stages of the pandemic, relatives were completely banned from visiting due to the desperation of trying to control the spread of Covid-19. One family were so concerned, they took their elderly relative out of the nursing home because they feared for their relatives life. This family were reported to the police for taking their relative, they were then followed down the motorway and stopped by the police. I don't remember what the outcome was but I remember seeing this with disbelief. I remember feeling so frightened for Mum, especially as I was solely responsible for keeping her safe. If anyone came to the house to do any work on the conservatory, I would ask them to do a Covid antigen test before they entered. We had these tests very early in the pandemic because we were on the Covid testing list with work. Although, Mum was very vulnerable to catching Covid, we never wore a mask when we were around her because Mum relied on lip reading due to her poor hearing.

In August 2020, I was exhausted and truly needed a break so that I could recharge and have a rest from being woken every two hours during the night. Sharon also needed a break and a week off work. So I did some research and found a lovely nursing home nearby that seemed to have strict Covid controls. Some nursing homes had point blankly refused to admit Covid patients from hospital and some had their own strict Covid restrictions. These nursing homes faired better on the number of deaths and managed to keep their residents safe. I went to visit the nursing home prior to Mum going in for a week's respite. The building was old but very comfortable and it looked like a hotel so it would be a break for Mum as well. I told Mum that she could go on holiday at the same time as we did. Mum seemed happy with this. I packed a small suitcase for her. I reassured Mum that it was only for a week. Myself and Sharon went along with her to settle her in. I took everything she needed including her Sherry and her favourite glass for her night cap. She was paired up with another lady who had recently been admitted to the nursing home. They were both to be kept separate from the other residents as a precaution for everyone. I thought this was a very practical and sensible approach to preventing the possible spread of Covid. The staff were all lovely and Mum looked content as I walked away with a slight feeling of guilt.

Andrew and me like British holidays in the form of cycling or walking. We do at least one active holiday per year. In 2018 we had cycled Lands' End to John O'Groats and each year we do either a week or a fortnight of walking. We had walked many long distance walks such as the Coast to Coast and some of the National trails including The Cotswold Way, The Cleaveland Way and The Pembrokeshire Way to name a few.

We decided to start the South West Coast Path but to do it in sections. Unlike Raynor Winn and Moth in the Salt Path, we liked a bit of luxury and preferred to stay in Bed and Breakfast, Pubs or Bunk Houses when we did these holidays rather than camping. I suppose you could say we are not purists and we couldn't take a lot of time off work or time away from home because of Mum and the horses. I hadn't read Raynor Winn's book at this time but I had read the book Travels With Boogie: 500 Mile Walkies as well as Boogie Up the River by Mark Wallington. Since reading the book 500 Mile Walkies, I had always wanted to walk the South West Coastal Path. Two good friends of ours had also walked the South West Coastal Path and they said it was the best walk they had ever walked. So it was on our bucket list of walks to do. Our plan to walk any longer than a week was scuppered by needing to get back for Mum. For us to go away it takes a few logistics but we organised someone to care for the horses for the week whilst we were away. I usually like to complete a walk in one continuum and I often refer to myself as a 'Starter & Finisher' from Belbin's role models. However, Covid was making a lot of people reassess what was important and in some ways people were becoming more relaxed as they were taking on the 'Don't sweat the small stuff' approach to life. My thoughts were that it doesn't matter if we don't walk it in one go as long as we enjoy every minute of what we do walk and we can look forward to coming back next year and so on. This was also Bowie's holiday as he also needed a rest from his caring duties. Bowie had been taking his caring responsibilities very seriously but now it was time for him to have some fun and freedom.

When we go on walking holidays we normally travel to the start destination by a combination of trains, buses or taxi's. Then we would walk every day until the end of the week and then we would travel home using public transport. However, our plans had to be changed as a lot of places were still shut because of Covid. Also, we considered the train to be a high risk of contracting Covid. If we got Covid, it would affect being able to collect Mum on our return so we decided to take the car and relay it along the walk using either taxis or the local bus service. We travelled down the M5 and stopped at a service station for a toilet break. I walked into the service station communal area to look for the toilet and I was shocked of how busy it was. There were hundreds of people all heading south for a holiday, the place was packed and inside the ladies toilets the hand driers were blowing, potentially spreading the virus by blowing it into the air. People were not allowed to travel abroad due to the Covid restrictions so it seemed that everyone was heading for Cornwall and Devon. We left quickly and carried on our journey. We were concerned that the whole area where we were walking would also be packed but once we started out on the coast path, it was nice and quiet. We started our walk at Minehead in Somerset which is the start of the South West Coast Path and we walked for four days along the coastal path. It was just the tonic we desired, just being in the open, breathing in the sea air and having the sounds of the sea all around us is exactly what we needed. Bowie loved it too, dogs love to travel and feel that they have purpose. Bowie's fur would part in the wind and he would stick his nose in the air to catch the smells. We couldn't continue along the path after four days because a lot of B&B's had shut down because of the pandemic. So we drove down to Polperro in Cornwall, where we had hired a cottage for a few days. Polperro is a beautiful tiny quaint seaside village which is more or less free of traffic due to its narrow streets. It has a small harbour and lots of unique gift shops. Our cottage was an old fisherman's cottage which was a great base to come back to after a long walk and some great food in the local pub. We walked for another three days in that area along the coast. The Somerset and Cornwall coast lines are very different but both just as enjoyable. Walking along the coast line from Polperro in either direction is pretty tough with lots of ascents and descents. We had been very lucky with the weather that week, the sun was shining and shimmering off the water. The end of our holiday seemed to arrive too soon. Even though we were walking every day, we had found it relaxing and we had been able to switch off from the chaos of our busy lives, work pressures as well as being able to distance ourselves from Covid for a few days. It had been like swimming under water for a long time and coming up for air, we were now ready to return home.

It was time to return to work, pick up Mum and settle back into our usual routine. When I went to pick up Mum, she was in great spirits, she was feeling well and in the belief that she had been on holiday. She told us stories about her stay, the people were friendly, the food was good but she was glad to see us and to be coming home. There were no negative comments about the workers which was a surprise and strangely slightly disappointing. One of the care staff asked me 'Who is Alan? And 'You must be Isabel, we have heard all about you'. Mum said her goodbyes and off we went. I was really impressed with the nursing home for keeping Mum safe and it gave me confidence that we could go on holiday again as Mum was relaxed and content. The trouble with having a break from living with someone with dementia is that after a couple of hours all that peace and relaxation is forgotten. Mum was still asking,

'Have you seen Alan?'

She had forgotten that he had died and this brought the familiar pain back into my chest. Bowie was thrilled to see Mum and the routine of ear tickling recommenced. I was hoping after such a great response in the nursing home, Mum would be more settled. However, in the evening Mum was still very restless and night time sleep was disturbed with the familiar jingle.

When we finally kiss goodnight
How I'll hate going out in the storm
But if you'll really hold me tight
All the way home I'll be warm

And the fire is slowly dying
And, my dear, we're still goodbying
But as long as you'd love me so
Let it snow! Let it snow, and snow!

I had forgotten about the Christmas song jingle in the week we were away but I was soon reminded. I would hear that jingle and before I really knew what was happening I would throw my legs out of bed, be moving towards the stairs, running down the stairs half asleep. How I never fell on the stairs I will never know as I was just acting on autopilot. Then I would be helping Mum back to her room, assisting her to the toilet before tucking her up in her comfy chair and getting her a drink and a snack before going back to bed myself. I would sleep for a few hours before the jingle sounded and exactly the same routine would follow. This could happen up to six times a night. Within a few weeks of being back home it felt like I hadn't been away.

In October 2020, Covid restrictions came back in the form of a Tier system which no one really understood. There was another Lockdown from 5th November until 2nd December 2020. It was Mum's 85th birthday on 6th December 2020 which was pleasant and low key. Mum's grandchildren and great grandchildren stayed away because of the restrictions but also because they didn't want to increase the risk of Mum contracting Covid. Before we went to work in the morning, we would get up at 6am, I would sort Mum out with a wash and breakfast and then Andrew and I would go out to feed, muck out and turn out the horses. We would race back in to the house, get changed ready for work. Sharon would arrive and then we would go to work. Ashley had now returned to live in London. At 5pm, we would return home, relieve Sharon from her duties, go out to care for the horses and then make our evening meal. We were all living in this regular routine which I think helped Mum cope with the challenges of living with dementia. The same routine each day kept Mum as settled as she could be in the daytime. The Alzheimers was taking its toll on Mum, you could see that she was deteriorating faster than what I had imagined or read up on. The anxiety she experienced was extreme especially because she was constantly looking for Dad. She believed he hadn't come home which was very distressing for her. She was looking much older and frail. Christmas 2020, was a quiet and relaxed one because we stayed at home, Allister came to see Mum but otherwise we didn't have any visitors but we were relatively happy in our little Bubble.

⸺◄❰❱►⸺

Chapter 16

Get Out

In January 2021, there was another Lockdown until the 2nd February 2021. This didn't really affect Andrew and I because we had grown accustomed to being at home without visitors. However, it did mean that Mum didn't see the rest of the family and because of this she was becoming more isolated. She was forgetting who people were because she did not see them anymore. She was beginning to forget who her grandchildren were and she hadn't got a clue about her great grandchildren anymore. She was unable to visualise them. This isolation was very damaging to Mum's memory. We noticed that Mum was getting increasingly agitated in the evening. She wanted to leave the house and would say,

'Right, I'm off now, Alan will be wondering where I am'

We tried everything to persuade her and prevent her from leaving by any method apart from physical restraint. We told her it was too cold to go outside and that it was dark, unsafe, raining but nothing would convince her to want to stay. She just had the burning desire to go. We tried distraction methods but they only lasted a few minutes. I thought back and remembered what we did with Grandma Beech, which was to let her go. So I thought it was worth a try but quite a risk to her from falling.

'OK, Mum, I think you should stay because it's very late but if you must go, let's get you wrapped up against the cold'

I helped her put on a warm coat and Smurf hat and then I would help her exit the front door. We would watch her walk up the path to the gate. Sometimes she would venture further but then before she got to the top of the drive she always turned around and came back.

'I will go in the morning! You are right it's a bit late'

'OK, let's get you ready for bed then and get you a sherry'

Mum's behaviour became more extreme and agitated in the evening. It seemed like she wanted an argument. I couldn't work out whether she was seeking an argument or just being naughty. There was no help and no one to ask why she was behaving this way. Andrew found it particularly difficult to deal with, especially as it wasn't his mother but also because all we wanted was peace and Mum seemed to want to fight every evening. This was not in Mum's control though and the phenomena is called 'Sundowning'. Sundowning is very common in dementia. Dementia UK describe Sundowning as a term used for changes in behaviour that occur in the evening, around dusk. Some people who have dementia experience a growing sense of agitation or anxiety at this time. This was definitely the case for Mum. Sundowning came as quite as surprise as we had never experienced this before first hand. Sundowning often makes the person with dementia feel very strongly that they are in the wrong place or in my Mum's case, that we were! Mum wanted us to leave. Sundowning may cause the person to say that they want to go home, even if they are at home. Mum never had an issue with being at Lapwing Farm, she loved it there and was very settled. She never seemed to miss her old house. However, she did want to go home to find Dad. She was always looking for Alan. She would sometimes refer to him as 'My Husband' rather than Alan. She may have forgot who other people were but she never forgot Dad.

There were times when Mum didn't know who we were though and this was becoming more frequent. Sometimes, she would think that we were the managers of a hotel that she was staying in and she would criticise the service she was receiving.

'Well this hotel is rubbish, it's a wonder it's still open. I don't know how you two are still in business, the service is rubbish'.

'This is not a hotel Mum, it's our home'

'How do you stay in business when there's no one else staying here, just me'

'This is not a hotel Mum, it's our home'

'Huh'

'I'm your daughter Isabel, don't you know me'

'Of course and that's why I'm worried. You and Andrew have set this all up and you must have spent a lot of money. What are you going to do if you don't get more guests.'

'This is not a hotel Mum, it's our home'

She would ignore any reasoning particularly in the evenings. This agitation started to escalate and she sometimes showed other signs of Sundowning which included pacing, shouting, arguing or becoming totally confused about everything. Sometimes I would become Thelma. As the evening approached, Andrew and I started to dread what was coming as you could see her mood changing and we knew we were in trouble. On one occasion I went for a soak in the bath and then I heard a commotion in the hall.

'Get out of my house!!'

'This is not your house, it belongs to me and Isabel'

'Don't talk such rubbish, me and Alan bought this house years ago and you are just abusing it'

'This is not your house'

'Get out of my house, I won't tell you again, just wait until Alan comes home'

Although Andrew knew that Mum couldn't help it and she was confused, he used to get drawn in to these petty arguments. Needless to say, I didn't stay soaking in the bath for long. By the time I had come downstairs, Andrew was exasperated and Mum would be fuming. One day she picked up a huge oak dining table and threw it out of her way. Her strength was impressive and quite surprising.Andrew and I would then start arguing with each other because he had made her worse.

'What am I supposed to do when she is asking me to leave my house.'

'Don't rise to it, you just make her worse.'

'That is easier said than done.'

In the evenings, we sometimes tried to watch a film but it would be near enough impossible to concentrate. I would have to get up and go to Mum about thirty times during the film as Mum would be constantly be calling or trying to get into the fridge. It would seem like attention seeking behaviour and I could feel myself becoming irritated. However, sometimes and on the odd occasion the following morning she would have a minute or two of clarity.

'I was bloody daft last night, why didn't you hit me over the head with a hammer, bloody crackers'.

'Its OK Mum, you were confused, you thought you were in a hotel.'

'Bloody crackers'

Then five minutes later she was back in chaos and confusion.

The next few months passed slowly with a day-in day-out routine. The workmen continued to work on the new conservatory which provided Mum with some entertainment with her critical remarks. The workmen tolerated the abuse with mild amusement. It was quite a busy house with Mum and the carers but the workmen always tried to work outside and were very respectful. They realised that Mum was a vulnerable person who they had become fond of and who they wanted to protect from Covid. They were also willing to conduct Lateral Flow Covid tests to make sure that they were clear if they needed to enter the house.

Mum continued to mobilise on her own by walking around with the aid of a blue walker with wheels, it had a hidden compartment where she could put her handbag, it had brakes and a seat so if she became tired she could sit down. Mum continued to do a few little jobs around the house like brass cleaning and vegetable preparation. She helped me with tack cleaning and loved coming down to the stables where she could spend time with horses. Mum was always content when she came down to the stables as the horses relaxed her. She would come down wearing her blue hat and she was always accompanied by Bowie on his lead. Bowie never pulled her and seemed to accept his caring responsibilities. I didn't mind Mum coming down to the stables unless I was riding as that could prove disastrous if she needed the toilet or if Mac spooked at her blue hat. If it was a cold day, I could set her up in the tack room, next to the heater and in the summer she would sit outside in the sunshine.

Next to the stables is the larger one of our two ponds. Mum used to enjoy sitting next to the pond and watching the activities of the wildlife on the pond. In March 2021, the pond was full of life and a pair of Canadian Geese were back, sitting on their nest in the usual position on a little island in the middle of the pond. They looked like the same pair who had been attending for mating and nesting since we moved in but we couldn't be sure. Canadian geese are very common in the UK. It has been noticed that they now breed in very small waterbodies particularly small lakes, meres or ponds. This was certainly true on our pond. The pair would noisily argue and stand their ground against other Canadian Geese until eventually there were just the two of them remaining. Canadian Geese don't seem to be bothered by humans being close even when breeding. This was definitely true of our pair. They didn't even bother about Bowie running around the pond. Bowie treats Canadian Geese like flying squeaky toys but as soon as they land, he loses interest and the chase is over. If other Canadian Geese fly over, he chases them, jumping in the air as if he is going to catch them but he never bothers with the two that are resident on the pond. The small island in the middle of the pond provides a safe haven for the large nest of eggs. The mother sits on the nest for weeks and the father swims around, waiting for the arrival of his babies. When the eggs eventually hatch, out would come the most beautiful fluffy goslings and within an hour they would all be swimming around on the pond. The mother would protect them from the front and the father would bring up the rear. The Mallard ducks, Coots and Moorhens would be chased away into the reeds. Approximately, twenty four hours later when the last gosling was strong enough to climb out of the steep sides of the pond, they would leave. Their mother would walk them through the horses field and take them across to the neighbouring Mill Pond. The Millpond is in a large field next door to our property, it is more like a small mere than a pond and there are hundreds of Canadian Geese living there. The strange thing is that about six to eight weeks later the same family of Canadian Geese return, usually with another family and all of their goslings as well. They all congregate together in their creche on our pond, it is fascinating to observe. The only time that the Canadian Geese annoy me is when they sit in the field and eat the horses grazing grass. The horses usually shoe them off their land though when they go out. It's a comical sight to see, a 17.1 hand high horse chasing the geese away with his head lowered to their level and his gangly legs going all over the place.

In the daytime at the weekends, there was peace at home and the pandemic provided a solace all of its own. There was an air of relative calmness until we went to work on a Tuesday. Once I had left for work, Mum would start to panic and Sharon would do her best to pacify Mum. Sometimes, the naughty behaviour and irrational episodes would get the better of Sharon. I would quite often get a phone call from a distraught Sharon.

'I don't know if I can do this anymore. Your Mum hates me'.

'She doesn't hate you Sharon, it's the dementia. She probably thinks you are someone else'.

By the time Sharon had gone back to Mum, her mood would have changed again. I was very aware that Sharon had not had any experience in care prior to caring for Mum, or with caring for old people anyway. Despite the care course and learning that Sharon was doing, she found it hard to rationalise that Mum could be so agitated, naughty and at times very difficult. Sharon would sometimes phone me up whilst I was at work to tell me that things were bad at home.

'Your Mum's left, I don't know what to do'.

'Let her go, she won't go far'

'But she has gone up the drive, what if she falls? What do you want me to do'

'Just let her go, if she falls, it's not your fault and it's a risk we will just have to take'

Then after a short while Sharon would phone me back,

'She has come back in now and she is alright again, calm now.'

Mum would quite often involve the builders.

'Help me, I'm in trouble, can you help me? Someone has stolen my train ticket'

Well the look on the lads faces was a picture, they were speechless. It was so random. Mum continued to gradually become more and more agitated which was particularly bad at night.

'That's it, I'm leaving'

'Go on then, but it's a long way to walk and its cold out there'

'Well I don't care I'm not staying with you two anymore, I'm going to jump in the 'Cut' and have done with it'

'There is no point doing that Mum, its only waist deep'

Mum had always threatened self-harm. As long as I could remember throughout the years, from time to time when she was not happy, she would threaten to jump in the 'Cut'. The 'Cut' is a Staffordshire name for canal. It seemed to be Mum's favourite threat of method for suicide. I even remember her saying it to my Dad when I was a child and I had cried believing that she really was going to do it. Although, it was always an empty threat, I had always wondered why she would say it. With these common outbursts and absolute chaos, the evenings were becoming intolerable as the Alzheimer's progressed and the Sundowning became worse.

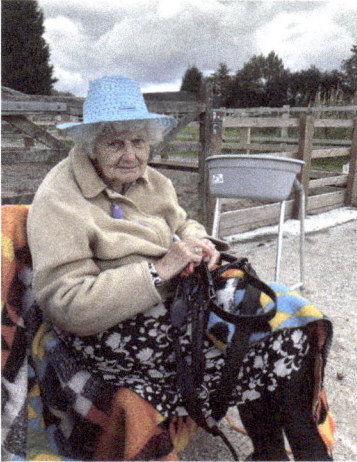

Mum, the Zimmer and
the Hat, the collie is not
far away

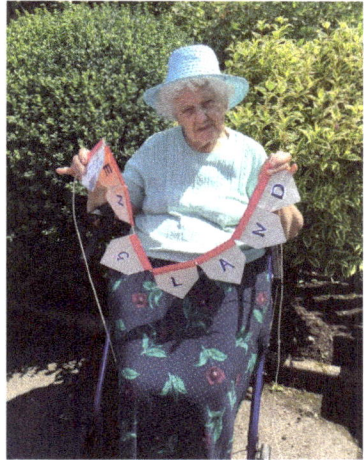

Mum wearing her
favourite blue hat

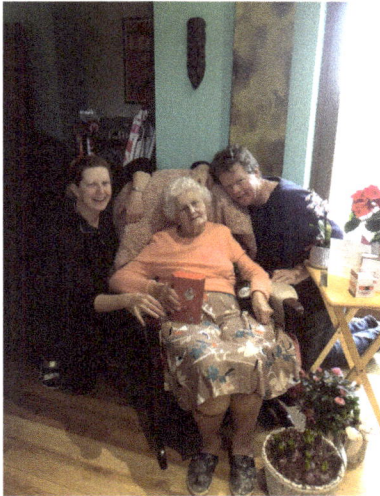

Allister, Mum and me on her birthday

Chapter 17

A Cry for Help

It was a long time in coming but eventually in April 2021 and after all the problems were solved with the foundations, the new oak room for Mum was completed. The days suddenly became peaceful, no more builders or electricians and no more hammering. We moved the sofas, the dining table and chairs and other bits and pieces of furniture back into the conservatory. The new oak room sat on the same footprint as the old conservatory but it gave the impression of being more spacious. The ceiling was slightly higher and there was a glass sky lantern in the roof which allowed lots of light into the room. The walls were painted in cream which complimented the oak beams. We got the chimney sweep out to check the chimney and then the log burner was refurbished. A carbon monoxide alarm was fitted for safety. The oak room was perfect and just as I had imagined it to be. It's large windows gave you the sensation of being outside, living amongst the wildlife. We placed Mum's rocking chair in a prime position, facing out over the garden. It was so tranquil for Mum, she could now sit in the rocking chair and was able to watch the antics of the wildlife. She could sit at the dining table and do her crafts or jigsaws with her carers. But most importantly, it was warm and dry. No more leaks which meant no more worry about her slipping and falling. This environment provided Mum with a much needed space which was peaceful. It was an area for calmness and it is what I had envisioned when she moved in. I had begun to worry that it would never be finished.

But the summer of 2021 was enjoyable, we would all sit in the conservatory together and just enjoy each other's company and the surroundings. On a hot day, the bi-folding doors could be opened so that a breeze entered the room which meant that the room could be kept cool and comfortable.

During the spring and summer of 2021, it was obvious that Mum was continuing to deteriorate and faster than what I had read or expected. Mum was taking a cocktail of drugs every day which were supposed to be trying to slow down the dementia. She took Donepezil, mainly for her Alzheimer's dementia. The psychiatrist had also mentioned when we visited him before Covid that he thought Mum may have a mixture of Alzheimer's and Vascular dementia. The Vascular type of dementia was never confirmed. The Donepezil is a Acetylcholinesterase inhibitor, it is supposed to slow the dementia by preventing an enzyme from breaking down a substance called acetylcholine in the brain, which helps nerve cells to communicate with each other. She also took a drug called Memantime, this was supposed to block the effects of an excessive amount of a chemical in the brain called glutamate. Glutamate is a neurotransmitter needed in the brain for learning, cognitive processing and memory. It is also an important mood regulator. Abnormally high levels of glutamate can increase a person's risk of certain neurological conditions, such as Alzheimer's disease. I wasn't sure if these drugs were helping Mum or not. How can you tell when you can see that the person is deteriorating anyway. But you wouldn't want to stop the medication because to do so was giving up, any help was hope. I researched online about the different stages of Alzheimer's and thought maybe Mum was in the middle stages of the disease. There are different scales which are just guides as everyone's dementia journey is unique to them. I did find the Global Deterioration Scale (CGS) / Reisberg Scale useful. I could safely say that Mum was at stage 6 by June 2021 which is when a person has severe cognitive decline. Stage 1 indicates a pre-dementia stage with no cognitive impairment, whereas Stage 7 is within the dementia diagnostics with very severe cognitive decline. Stage 7 is the final stage according to this scale. Calculating by using this scale was the only way that I could gage the deterioration. The deterioration seemed to be rapid compared to other people that I knew who had Alzheimer's though. What I found was extremely difficult is that there was no support available. There were no doctor appointments due to the pandemic. There were no further follow ups at the hospital in the memory clinic. I knew I was not the only person struggling to care for a relative at home with dementia but I did feel abandoned by the care system and there was no one to turn to due to the pandemic crisis. As soon as the word dementia or Alzheimers was mentioned, you could see the likelihood of help or support being shut down.

The daytimes could be quite enjoyable and sometimes mildly entertaining. However, the evenings continued to be extremely challenging with no relaxation or peace. The nights were a pattern of broken sleep and agitation. Mum was continually getting up and wandering about downstairs in the house. The movement sensor alarm next to my head would suddenly start up with the now mind numbing Christmas song 'Let it snow', even in the middle of a heat wave;

When we finally kiss goodnight
How I'll hate going out in the storm
But if you really grab me tight
All the way home I'll be warm
Oh, the fire is slowly dying
And, my dear, we're still goodbying
But as long as you'd love me so
Let it snow, let it snow, let it snow!

This song was brainwashing me into action, my legs would be on the move before my brain had registered what was happening or what I was doing. I was like one of Pavlov's dog acting on an automatic response. I was seriously suffering from sleep deprivation. I thought about changing the alarm's tune just to have some variety. I never bothered though as I used to quite like the song and even though it was repetitive it was strangely comforting and better than the other choices. I know if I ever hear that tune in the future, it will remind me of jumping out of bed and running down the stairs.

One night the movement sensor alarm went off and I raced down stairs. I could hear a lot of doors banging and commotion coming from Mum's bedroom. It was about the fifth or sixth time that night that I had been down to settle Mum. I was exhausted and at my wits end. I walked into her bedroom to find that she had been very busy. I looked at her as my brain fog began to clear, I could see she was fully dressed.

'What are you doing Mum, you are dressed?'

'Nowt, I'm just getting up'

'It's only 3am Mum, you need to get some sleep and so do I, I need to go to work in a few hours, let me help you get your nightie back on'

That's when I noticed that all of her clothes out of the wardrobe were piled in a big heap on the bed. I started to help Mum to remove one of the jumpers that she was wearing and then realised that she was dressed in at least six or seven layers of clothing.

'Are you cold?'

'No, why?'

'Oh Mum, what have you been doing, what are all of these clothes doing on the bed and why are you wearing six jumpers?'

I started to clear away the clothes and to put them back into the wardrobe. I put an item of clothing back onto a coat hanger and then something came over me that I had never experienced before. It was like a blind rage. I picked up the bundle of clothes off the bed and chucked them on top of Mum's head. Then I immediately came to my senses and burst into tears.

'What you done that for? You Peevish Bugger!'

'Oh Mum, I'm sorry, I'm just so tired'

'You want to get yourself to bed then, you have been busy at work, you should tell 'em' at work, it's not on. This nursing home is putting on you and you are the only person working here. You should complain!'

'Come on Mum, let me put these clothes away and let's get you settled down'.

This took me quite a while and then I dragged myself back to bed, where Andrew was happily snoring away, oblivious to all the commotion. How I envied him. The next morning I told Andrew that I had committed some sort of strange domestic abuse and of how ashamed I was. I told him that I was going to report myself as a safeguarding risk to Mum. I have been nursing for thirty plus years and this was the first time I had ever lost my patience. Andrew told me I was being too hard on myself and that I was bound to be affected by the lack of sleep. He couldn't help me with Mum either, for one reason he is not a carer but also because he couldn't take Mum to the toilet as it just would not be decent.

I knew I had to do something because I felt at my wits end. So I phoned the General Practitioner's surgery to ask for help and to report myself as a safeguarding risk. I put the request on the online triage form which was a new system since Covid. I wrote that I was sleep deprived and that I had chucked all of Mum's clothes on the top of her head. I wrote that I wasn't coping and that I thought Mum was a safeguarding risk. I was hoping for some help but I didn't know what that would look like. Anyway, my online triage form must have triggered a Safeguarding alert and I got a phone call very quickly. That's great I thought, someone is going to help me. I was a little worried that they would take Mum away from us. However, on reflection, I don't think that would ever happen especially with her having Alzheimer's dementia. There were no hospital beds anyway and dementia seems like a poor mans choice of illness. No one seemed to be interested in Alzheimers patients, they were seen as a burden to society. Anyway, I received a phone call from the doctors surgery. The person who phoned me had a very gentle and soft voice with an empathetic air to her tone.

'Hello, my name is Jane and I am a Social Prescriber'

'Oh hello, that's great, what sort of help can you provide'

'I can talk to you'

'Talk to me?'

'Yes, tell me about what you are struggling with?'

'I am just so tired, Mum gets me up every night about six to eight times a night. I am exhausted! Is there any respite care available or are there any care givers that could come and give me an hours rest?'

'No we don't provide that sort of service, I am here for you though, to talk'

'In the past, when my parents looked after their parents and because that was seen as saving the NHS money, they used to get a two week break for respite care'

'There isn't any respite offered these days. Social prescribing can really help you though'

Meanwhile I could hear Mum flushing the toilet in her bathroom. This made me anxious because Mum was no longer capable of going to the toilet on her own. She may have wet herself or worse. She may be putting lots of toilet paper or incontinence pads into the toilet which would block the toilet or it would cause havoc with our septic tank.

'Look I know you mean well but I need physical help. I'm sorry but I need to go as I can hear Mum in the toilet and I need to go and supervise her and to help her'.

'OK, well lets reschedule and I will call you next week'.

'I don't know if this is going to cause me more stress to be honest'

'Well I am here for you if you need me'.

'Ok, thank you'.

I didn't want to appear ungrateful but talking was not going to be of any help to me. It would be too difficult to give up the time to talk about my problems and I just could not see it helping either. It was a physical presence that I needed rather than talking and anyway I could talk to Andrew whenever I wanted to.

One weekend, my brother, Allister did offer to come and sit with Mum whilst we went out for a few hours. So we booked to go out for a meal. I thanked him very much and told him that we would only be an hour or so. He had brought Mum some fruit, she had always loved fruit but her stomach no longer tolerated it.

'Please don't give Mum that fruit as it will upset her stomach'.

'She will be alright it's only a small amount and it's healthy'

'No, please don't. It doesn't suit her these days.'

Off we went for a meal, it was nice to go out on a 'date night'. I made an effort and put some nice clothes and make up on. We went to a local gastro pub for a lovely meal. We were gone for approximately an hour and a half. On our return, Allister looked concerned.

'I think Mum has had an accident in her toilet whilst you were out. I haven't been to investigate, she was in there for ages but I have made sure she has washed her hands properly'.

'You didn't give her that fruit, did you?'

'Yes, but I thought she would be alright and she loved it'.

'I did tell you, Mum can't tolerate fruit anymore, it gives her terrible diarrhoea'.

I escorted Mum to her bathroom to assess the situation. Poor Mum had been incontinent of faeces and she had tried her best to clean herself up. She would have been very embarrassed to let Allister know and he would not have been able to cope to clean her up anyway. In her attempt to clean herself, she had managed to make more of a mess in the sink and on the towels. It took me an hour to get Mum showered and sorted out. Quite frankly, it wasn't worth the effort of going out. One of the carers at the weekend also made the mistake of not listening to me about the fruit either. Only on that occasion the carer had to deal with the consequences of not listening.

One of the grandchildren, Rob and his wife Sarah offered to have Mum over at their new house for a day out. At first, I was a bit reluctant to let Mum go as Rob would not be able to take Mum to the toilet. I was also worried in case a similar accident occurred at their house with the toilet situation. However, Rob reassured me that Sarah didn't mind and had looked after one of her elderly relatives, so I let Mum go out for the day. I prepared a bag with incontinence pads, wipes, gloves and waste bags similar to what I did when my son, Cameron was a baby. Rob picked Mum up and off she went for the day. I was a little apprehensive throughout the day but I need not of worried as they did an amazing job of looking after Mum and she had loved seeing her great grandchildren. This was the sort of help I needed. This gave me the idea to get in touch with a care agency and I booked a few evenings so that we could go out. This was great and the care staff were good but Mum couldn't really afford for us to do this very often as it was very expensive, costing £20 for 30 minutes. We only did use this service a few times but when we did it felt like a luxury.

Despite these mini relief breaks, I was still exhausted and felt suffocated by Mum's constant need to be with me. Andrew was also struggling with the evening agitation. We both really needed a break so that we could mentally relax. Covid was less of a risk now so we decided to go away for another week so that we could go walking. We feel that walking is the best type of mental relaxation. But first, I needed to find a nursing home that took people with Alzheimer's dementia for respite care. The nursing home that Mum had gone to the previous year couldn't cope with Mum's needs now due to the progression of the disease. I went onto the internet and searched for local nursing homes that take dementia patients. One jumped out at me because it was new and purpose built with dementia care in mind. This meant that it would be safe and it was probably very pleasant giving Mum the feel that it was a hotel and that she was also having a holiday. The nursing home was in Willaston which is close to Crewe and Nantwich, Cheshire. I telephoned them to make an enquiry. It did specialise in dementia and it only had a few residents because it had only just opened. I thought this may be perfect for Mum because she would get lots of attention. It also meant that low numbers of residents meant I didn't have to worry about her mixing with lots of other residents and contracting the dreaded Covid. So far Mum had not had Covid and that is the way that I wanted it to stay. I took Mum to have a look at the nursing home and we were shown around. It was a complete new build with a separate dementia unit upstairs which was completely secure but it did not give the impression of imprisonment. The upstairs area still had open outside areas as well as communal lounges. It looked and felt like a hotel and was really nice. There were only a handful of residents who all seemed pleasant. The risk of Mum contracting Covid was definitely going to be minimal and she would have more of less one to one care. It was also close enough for Allister and all of the grandchildren to be able to visit Mum. It all seemed perfect and in some ways too good to be true.

So we booked Mum in for a week's stay from 17th June 2021. We took Mum to the nursing home and settled her in and then off we went on holiday. The staff were lovely and they made Mum feel at home. Mum appeared to be content thinking she was in a hotel on a holiday. She seemed to appreciate and understand that we needed a holiday but maybe she was a bit tired of us too and wanted a break herself. We had arranged for the horses to be cared for whilst we were away. So off we went to Devon and then Cornwall. Andrew, me and Bowie walked for a week on the South West Coast Path, setting off from where we had walked the previous year. We did four days in Devon and three days in Cornwall again which was continuing the same pattern as before. We love walking and this break in the fresh air was just what we needed. It was a well-deserved rest for Bowie, well you couldn't really say rest as he never stopped. Being a Border Collie meant that his energy levels were always high. In the evenings though he used to relax. Bowie had settled into his role as a caring dog and he took his role very seriously as a protector. He did this in exchange for constant tickles. Mum was more concerned about missing Bowie than us when we went on holiday.

During Mum's stay at the nursing home for the week, she had settled really well and believed that she was in a guest house in Llandudno. Allister went to visit her regularly and they had an Afternoon Tea in the lounge on the ground floor. He was also able to wheel Mum out in a wheelchair and take her around the garden area. She was very content. The nursing home was a great find and all of the family were happy that we had found somewhere so good. The staff got to know her really well and they laughed at how outspoken and critical she was of the maintenance worker, some of the carers and fellow patients. When we went to collect her to bring her home, she greeted me with a big smile.

'Oh, am I glad to see you' she laughed out loud, 'they are all bloody crackers in here!'

'Shush, Mum, you can't say that'

'Of course you can, that women over there has led the staff a right merry dance, bloody cracker's, I tell you'

'Mum, stop saying that, come on let's take you home, Bowie is waiting for you'.

Mum's face lit up 'Oh I have missed my Bow'

Mum had remembered who Bowie was and at that moment she appeared to be totally lucid. Maybe this break was what Mum needed too. She had certainly seemed to enjoy herself and the nursing home matron and staff seemed lovely. We gave them a box of chocolates as a thank you with a promise to see them all again. The cost of this care was £1600.00 per week which seemed expensive but that was the going rate for dementia care. It did seem worth it though as she had really enjoyed herself and we had been able to have a lovely relaxing week. It also didn't seem to unsettle or disorientate Mum either. It felt like a Win, Win solution. We planned that we would book Mum in for a holiday at this nursing home a few times a year which would give us all the respite we needed. But at that cost we couldn't afford to do that too often and I was aware that I needed to ration Mum's money out as it needed to last her for the rest of her life. Looking after mum's money and making it last was a huge responsibility. Finding that nursing home was a huge relief though, we had found somewhere so good and it was like a five star hotel. Mum had always been so against nursing homes and considered them to be like the Workhouse, however, this was different and she seemed to have relished her time there. The staff at the nursing home seemed to genuinely like Mum. I was very happy that I had found somewhere so suitable.

Chapter 18

The Collapse

Mum was already packed up, the nurses had made sure she was ready so we all returned home. Bowie was thrilled to see Mum and greeted her with total affection, he was soon having his ears tickled. The routine of life returned to the sort of normality that we were used to. That was me looking after Mum for all her day to day needs, taking Aunty Pam her shopping on a Monday and working Tuesday to Friday. Sharon took over caring for Mum in the daytime, Tuesday to Friday with Karen and Debbie doing alternative weekends. This weekend help meant that I could ride my horses and go to horse shows without worrying about Mum. Now that we had a plan for further respite, the evenings seemed to be more manageable. Life was good.

Then one day when I was caring for Mum I noticed that she became very unresponsive and I could not get her to stand up. She became floppy like a rag doll. It was strange as she wasn't unconscious but she wasn't alert either. I took her temperature which was normal as was her blood pressure and pulse. I couldn't put my finger on what was wrong and causing this unresponsive episode. When you care for someone on a one to one basis and you are with them for long periods of time, you know when they just aren't quite right. I was just about to call the doctor when she started to come around and within a few hours she was back to talking, eating and could walk to the toilet. That evening I got Mum ready for bed early, she was very sleepy and docile that evening but she had made a full recovery by the morning. As a nurse, I wondered whether she had a Transient Ischaemic Attack (TIA). These episodes called TIA's may also be called a "mini stroke" and they are caused by a temporary disruption in the blood supply to part of the brain. The disruption in blood supply results in a lack of oxygen to the brain. This can cause symptoms similar to that of a stroke, such as speech problems, visual disturbances and numbness or weakness in the face, arms and legs. The symptoms usually resolve themselves and there is little anyone can do about them. Anyway, Mum returned more or less to her normal self, so I never bothered calling the doctor as I knew that there was nothing that could be done. Following this episode, Mum became slightly less mobile and tended to sit for longer periods than she normally would. This was great for me in the evenings because I didn't have to keep getting up to settle Mum down again but it was concerning. Over the next few weeks, gradually, it became difficult to get Mum to walk to the car which meant that her visiting days of going out were limited.

There was a subtle change in Mum's wellbeing, she became more confused and muddled about everything. This made her more anxious. Most of the time she believed she was in a nursing home and would say,

'Thank you Nurse'

'Who am I? Mother'

'I know you, don't I?'

'Yes, I'm your daughter, Isabel, you live with me, Andrew and Bowie and you are safe'

'Of course, I do get muddled, you know'

On the days when Sharon was looking after Mum, Sharon wasn't coping very well with caring for Mum since her deterioration so we started doubling up the care with

Karen coming at the same time as Sharon for a few hours in the daytime. This allowed Sharon to nip out when she needed to care for her own animals. Sharon also used to fetch in my horses in from the field in the afternoon and she was now only able to do this if Karen was there. Mum was too anxious to leave on her own at this stage even for a few minutes. Mum was no longer able to go in Sharon's car to do errands such as collecting the horse feed for Sharon's horses or to go to the equestrian centre to watch the dressage. Mum really missed these trips, the change of scenery and the variety that the outings presented. The lack of freedom was also difficult for Sharon and she was finding being stuck at our house caring for Mum, very challenging now.

One day whilst I was at work, I got a phone call in the afternoon from Sharon saying that Mum was not well and that I should come home straight away. Karen and Sharon were both sitting with Mum.Andrew and I left work immediately and came home. Sharon and Karen were comforting Mum, holding her hand and reassuring her. Mum was again unresponsive but this time she was unconscious. This episode was much worse than the last one. She was in a collapsed slumped state in her chair. Her eyes were shut and she was totally unresponsive. I did her basic observations which were her temperature, blood pressure and pulse, all of these were unremarkable. I was just about to call for an ambulance when her eyes opened but I could tell that she wasn't really awake. She was still totally floppy, unresponsive to speech and was slumped in her chair. My opinion was that she had had a stroke or another TIA but this time it was more severe. I thanked Sharon and Karen and let them go home with a promise of an update once I had phoned the emergency services. So I phoned 999 and the call was answered. When you call 999, they ask what service you want and I told the person it was the ambulance service. I was put through straight away and asked whether the patient was breathing. I told them that she was breathing and then they asked me another thirty plus other questions. They go through a standard series of questions as part of their triage which I answered yes or no to. Eventually, I was allowed to speak and tell the ambulance triage person what had happened. I told the operator that my Mum had Alzheimers disease and that she had collapsed and was initially unconscious, that she was now semi-conscious, floppy and unresponsive. I could not believe what was said to me.

'I'm sorry but this is not a 999 call. This is not an emergency but we will get a doctor to call you within 4 hours'

I sat there in shock, that was the end of the call, just like that, dismissed! I could not believe that a person who is semi-conscious, who may have had a stroke would not be an emergency call. I was kicking myself for telling them about the Alzheimers as I believe this impacted on the decision making through the triage process. I am also aware that the ambulance service was stretched and that Covid patients were bed blocking hospital beds but this decision just seemed wrong on any level. To actually not treat a semiconscious patient as an emergency. I felt hopeless and distressed but I didn't believe that I could do anything about it. I certainly couldn't move her or get her into a car to take her to the hospital myself because she was semi-conscious. Andrew and myself tried to get Mum to stand but her arms were limp. We just waited for the doctor to call but no doctor came or phoned either. Four hours came and went by without a phone call. After approximately six hours, I did receive a phone call from a nurse practitioner. I confirmed that Mum was still semi-conscious and that I was very concerned about her. Mum was totally floppy and we could not move her from the chair that she was sitting in as we did not have anyway of lifting her up. I told the nurse practitioner that Mum was incontinent of urine and potentially faeces' and that she had been stuck in the same position, in the char now for six hours and I was really concerned that she may develop a pressure sore. This had no impact on the urgency for action. I was told that a nurse practitioner would call in to see Mum and that she was now on the call out list. I tried to tell them that I thought Mum had had a TIA or stroke but the nurse practitioner did not consider or respect my knowledge, experience or specialist nurse qualification. I just could not believe how Mum was just being disregarded. I kept thinking that Mum had helped other people whenever they needed it and she had paid her national insurance all of her life and when she needed help, there was none. I tried to rationalise this diabolical lack of care by reminding myself that the NHS was in a direr way with Covid. This lack of concern for Mum brought it home to me of how bad things had become in the NHS. No one would come to help us, it was so saddening. Mum was just discarded by the 999 services and I was left trying to maintain Mum's airway and dignity for hours. I felt so depressed by this! What had become of the NHS to neglect someone in need like this. I would have taken Mum to hospital myself but we couldn't move her. I sat with Mum for 14 hours and eventually Mum started to come around. I was desperate to move Mum because of the high risk of pressure sores. When she was responsive enough and with the help of Andrew, I managed to get Mum to transfer into her wheelchair so that I could move her to take her to her room. Later I managed to transfer her on to a commode which I had got for emergencies. I washed Mum, changed her wet underwear and incontinence pad. Luckily her skin was red but intact. Mum managed a few sips of water. It was obvious that she was coming around albeit very slowly. After another 2 hours, so 16 hours in total since my 999 call, there was a knock at the door. A nurse practitioner came in, not a doctor as initially promised. The nurse took Mum's temperature which was normal and then she stuck a urinalysis stick in Mum's incontinence pad and diagnosed a urine infection. This was a false diagnosis in my opinion which I tried to explain. Mum had always had a mild urine infection since she had experienced bladder problems following a prolapse many years ago and she took a daily low dose of antibiotic. I told the nurse that Mum's urine was no different and that was not the cause of her collapse. The nurse would not listen and the fact that I was a qualified nurse had no influence on her either.

'Well, she looks alright now, so here is a prescription for a course of antibiotics. If she has any further problems phone 111 or 999 if she collapses'

'Well, I already tried that last night, 16 hours ago'

'We are very busy'

The nurse practitioner spent about 5 minutes with Mum and then she was gone within a few minutes, leaving me feeling irrelevant, angry and dismayed. Unfortunately, I was also convinced that the behaviour and dismissive approach to Mum was caused by me mentioning her Alzheimers diagnosis. I thought maybe they believed that I was trying to get Mum into a ward on the NHS. This is what used to be known as dumping, when a relative no longer wants to care for a relative, they get them admitted into A&E. This was not the case at all with me, I wanted Mum to stay with me where she was safe but I did think that Mum needed some further investigations and not to be dismissed as she was.

After a few days, Mum seemed to have made a reasonable recovery but it had terrified the carers and now Sharon was concerned whether this may happen again. I was also very aware that the carers would not manage to move Mum with a hoist, even if we had one due to inexperience and lack of space. I don't think Mum would have coped very well with being hoisted either. Mum had collapsed twice now in a matter of a few weeks with the second one being much worse than the first. The emergency services refusing to come out did not help my concerns. I was very worried that this was going to become a regular occurrence that none of us could deal with at home. I was certainly not willing to leave Mum sitting in urine for 16 hours again because there was no help available. It was obvious that some difficult decisions needed to be made. Andrew and I talked it over with Allister and we came up with a three month plan to move Mum into the nursing home in Willaston permanently. Afterall, she had loved it there, the family liked it, it was easy for the family to visit and the care seemed good.

Andrew and me were planning another holiday. We had planned to go away for a week on 24th August, 2021. So the plan we came up with was to let Mum go into the nursing home again for another week so that she became more familiar with her surrounding and with the staff. She would then come home for another two months before moving her into the nursing home permanently. This would give all of the career three months' notice to find other work, which I thought was fair. It would also give us another opportunity to make sure that this was the right nursing home for Mum. This was an extremely difficult decision for me to make and I was completely torn in two. Mum's welfare was the most important thing to consider and I wanted her to stay with me. However, she was deteriorating and it would be impossible to manage if she kept collapsing or having TIA's which is what I firmly believed these episodes were. I tried to discuss the decision with Mum, I wasn't sure whether she understood what I was telling her but she did seem to accept what I was saying. Since the last episode of being semi-conscious for whatever reason, Mum just seemed quiet and accepting of anything. All of the bad evening behaviour had stopped, she just seemed placid and passive now. It was obvious that Mum's condition had changed and entered a different phase. There was no one from the medical profession to make an opinion on what was happening but change was definitely afoot.

After discussing the plan with the carers, everyone seemed to understand and accept that this was for the best. The carers were upset as they had cared for Mum for a long time now and they were attached to her funny ways. Sharon said that she thought it was for the best as she was finding caring for Mum very difficult now she wasn't as mobile. The plan was agreed for the three month transition period. However, the next day, sadly Sharon came and told me that she would look after Mum until her first nursing home week for respite but I would have to find someone else to look after Mum for the last two months. This left me with a major dilemma; without the care in the day, I would have to finish work and I couldn't afford to do that. Finding a carer just for two months didn't seem very achievable either. Also, without the care structure in the week, the weekend care would have to stop. Therefore the plan had to change, Mum would have go into the nursing home permanently on 24th August, 2024.

The next few weeks were busy with the preparation of moving Mum into the nursing home. This included choosing her a nice room. Me, Mum and Allister went to visit to pick a room for Mum. She chose a spacious room which was close to the nursing station and there was a balcony so that she would be able to go outside and she could even have a bird feeder out there. It all seemed to be very exciting and Mum was completely calm about it. However, I was all churned up inside as I had always promised Mum that I would look after her in her old age and I had also promised Dad that I would care for Mum after he had gone. I felt like I was failing and letting them both down somehow.

Before Mum went to stay in the nursing home, I thought it was important for Mum to see Uncle George, her brother. I managed with some difficulty to get Mum in the car and took her to see George. I explained to him and my cousin Christopher that I believed that this would be the last time that they would see each other. George was not that well himself so he was unlikely to be able to visit Mum in the nursing home. This visit was a heart wrenching and moving event. My Uncle George sat in his wheelchair looking frail, he had lost a lot of weight recently and he looked half the man he used to be. This strong brave man that used to be a Queen's Guard. He was now confined to a wheelchair because he only had one leg. He had had to have one leg amputated a few years ago. Mum sat next to him, also looking frail and lost. She was intensely looking up into his face as if seeking out that connection that only a brother and sister may have. They had lived through the second world war, had seen many modern inventions and had shared loss. They had once been young and vibrant, they had shared secrets and life events. As I sat with the two of them, they looked lost and grasped each other's hands in a strong embrace for a long time. I could see that they both knew what was happening, that this was the last time they would ever see each other. They knew that life had given them many years but it had now taken away some dignity, memories and physical capability. They knew that they hadn't got long left on the earth and it was their time soon. They were aware that they were in their last throws of life, that the end was nearing. They handled this knowledge and this last farewell with that great British stiff upper lip that their generation were accustomed to. They said their goodbyes like they were expected to, bravely. They didn't have to say it out loud and there were no spoken words to confirm what they knew. Usually, Uncle George would say 'Don't leave it so long, next time' but he just waved goodbye with a tear in his eye. I had explained to Mum why we were visiting George but I wasn't sure if she truly understood. However, despite the Alzheimers, I could see that Mum completely understood the magnitude of this visit.

I also took Mum on one last memory trip to where she had lived for most of her adult life, in Alsager. We drove around the familiar roads, past where me and my brother were born, past the school where she had worked and then onto her last house. We stopped the car so that she could speak to her old neighbours and of course I arranged for Mum's great friend, Thelma Bickerton to come to visit our home before Mum went to live in the nursing home. Thelma tried to reassure me that I had done all I could do and told Mum that she would visit her in the new posh and newly built nursing home. Thelma joked that Mum would have them all sorted out there in no time. The sadness of this decision was weighing heavily on my heart and I could not escape the feeling of guilt.

⦿

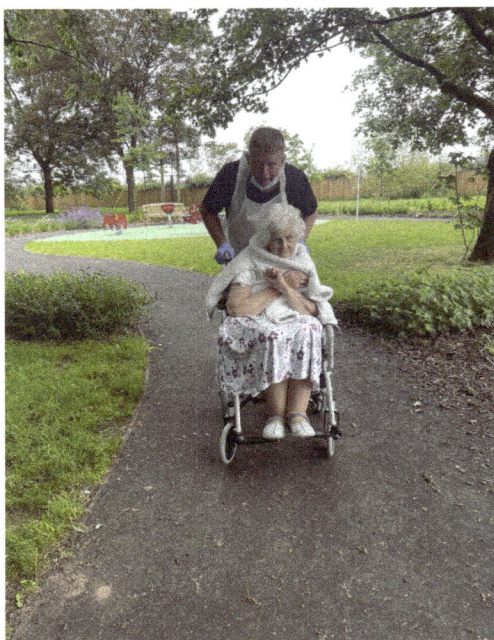

Allister visiting Mum at the nursing home

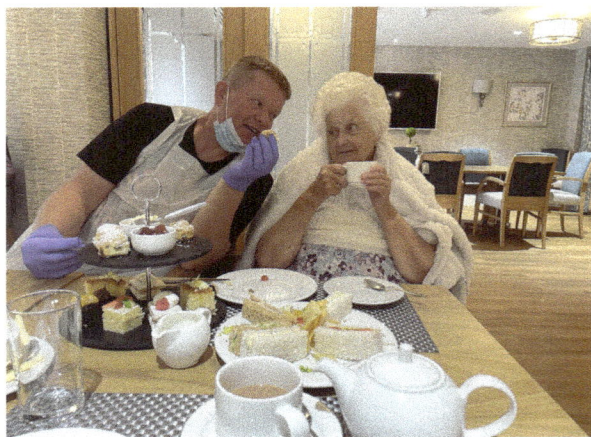

Allister and Mum enjoying afternoon tea at the nursing home

Chapter 19

The Nursing Home

I spent the next few weeks preparing Mum for when she moved to the nursing home. We decided together what she would take out of her room. What was the most disconcerting matter for me was her total acceptance of the situation. She seemed so placid about it all. This was not the Mum that I knew and loved, she had never been a placid person. Mum had brain washed me ever since I was a young child that it was my duty to care for her in her old age. So I found this acceptance very difficult to deal with. I was concerned that she may have just given up on life or that the possible TIA's had caused a profound change in her. I was also struggling with my own demons, worrying that I was doing the wrong thing. I was very mindful and concerned that the nursing home was very expensive. People with dementia have to pay more money because the demands are more on the nursing staff and there is supposed to be a higher ratio of nurses or carers to patients because of these additional demands. I had worked out that with Mum's money left over from the house sale and with paying the nursing home £1600.00 per week, her money would last approximately 12 months. So my grave concern and question is what would happen when her money had run out. Would she be asked to move out and to go in a council funded nursing home. I did not have a problem with council funded nursing homes as the care should and could be as good as a private nursing home. But we couldn't access one now and I didn't want her to have to be moved again. It was the moving from one place that she thought of as home to another place that was worrying me. Afterall, she had already moved out of her home and into ours and now I was moving her to a nursing home. Moving Mum when she was so confused and trying to rationalise her surroundings would surely have a negative effect on her cognitive functioning. Once she had run out of money, surely they would not ask her to move again but at the end of the day they were a private business. I did ask the nursing home about this and I didn't feel confident that they wouldn't ask her to move out. They did explain that there is some sort of top up but I didn't understand it at all. I was worried that if they asked her to move out when she had no money left , it would cause a lot of upset for her. She would be settled and believed it to be her home. I had raised this query with the nursing home again but I didn't get a clear answer. They tried to explain about the means to top up on the government allowance. I never really understood what this actually meant and they couldn't give me a satisfactory answer as they said it would depend on many factors. I asked if it meant that me and my brother would be expected to pay the additional money which was approximately £500 to £600 per week. They told me that yes, that was sometimes the case. I asked them what would happen if we could not afford that. There was not a straight forward answer to any of the questions so this was a major concern for me.

The week before Mum's departure, I labelled all of her clothes with permanent marker pen, just like she had done for me when I went to school many years ago. The day soon came around for Mum to go to live in the nursing home. So on 20th August 2021, I took Mum in the car and helped her to settle into her new surroundings. Again she seemed content. She told me that she could not have wished for a better daughter. This upset me more than if she had said something critical and it racked me full of guilt. I carefully unpacked her bag of clothes and put them away in the wardrobe neatly. I put the Croft Original sherry bottle and Mum's special sherry glass on the sideboard. I placed her toiletries and her prescribed Incontinence pads into her own bathroom. She had a nice set up and she was able to walk around her room with her walker, she could look out onto her balcony or she could wander out into the corridor and go to the communal lounge. The nursing home was a bit busier than it was on her last stay, they now had approximately twenty residents in the sixty bedded nursing home. There were a mixture of men and women wandering around, some had severe late stage dementia but there were a few residents that were able to have a conversation. Although, Mum was in the later stages of Alzheimers, she loved to talk and was very sociable so Mum would have some company. After a few hours in the nursing home I decided to leave Mum and she waved me goodbye. I went to leave three times before returning again as I just wanted to make sure she was alright. The nurse in charge could see that I was having difficulty leaving her and reassured me that she would be fine and that I could phone up later to check if she had settled. I felt so torn and I had a feeling of dread. It seemed easier to leave Mum when it was just for respite care, this felt too permanent. I finally dragged myself away, told Mum that I was going on holiday for a week and that I would come and see her on my return and that Allister would come to visit her over the next few days.

Once I had left, I tried to shake off the guilt and leave it behind me.Andrew and I went on the holiday that we had planned. This time we were taking Bowie with us for a week of enjoying the beautiful Snowdonia countryside. We had planned some mountain walking and some horse riding. We also took Mac (my horse) with us to Snowdonia Riding Stables for some schooling with our friend Melissa. Schooling is the name given for teaching the horse in a discipline that they are working on, in Mac's case it is dressage. I would be having some dressage lessons with Mac from Melissa and on other days we would go walking up the mountains. On the days when we were walking, Melissa would school Mac for me. Aine (Andrew's horse) didn't like going away from home so a friend was looking after her at home. Once we had dropped Mac off and settled him into his new home for the week, we went to find our accommodation. We were staying in a chalet in Waunfawr which is a beautiful small village and community, just outside Caernarfon in the Snowdonia National Park, Gwynedd, in Wales. The pine chalet was perfect, quiet and remote, just what we needed for a relaxing break.

That week the weather was kind to us and the sun was shining. We did a couple of walks, one up my favourite mountain, The Glyder's and another one up Carnedd Dafydd. We also fitted in a visit to our favourite area on Anglesey which is Newborough Beach and forest. We even went on a mountain hack with a few of the riding school horses and ponies to the shoulder of one of the lower mountains. Andrew was riding one of the riding school horses and I was on Mac. Mac did look a bit out of place amongst the ponies but he loved it. He stumbled over the rocks where the ponies were foot sure and he got a bit over excited on the mountain and bucked me off. I had to find a rock where I could climb back on but the fall on to moorland heather was soft so no harm was done. Snowdonia riding stables in Waunfawr is a gem, great horses and ponies who are well looked after and there are fantastic and knowledgeable riding instructors. The ponies and horses are so honest and really look after people. This area is one of my favourite places in the UK and the scenery is amazing. There are lots of outdoor activities you can do there such as walking and climbing and it is close to Anglesey where there are beautiful beaches. We always find walking a great therapy especially for sorting out conflicts which may be going on in your own head. I always feel like I can sort out my life within a few days of walking. I return to normal life following a few days walking knowing what I want to do and I always have a clearer vision. Horse riding is also very therapeutic for me. When I ride a horse I can only think about the movement of the horse and the surrounding environment. I find this very relaxing. We really enjoyed this holiday in North Wales. Once the break was over and we had returned home, sorted the animals out, we went to visit Mum and we took Bowie with us.

On our arrival, Mum was sitting in the corridor on a chair where she could watch everyone pass by. A pleasant charge nurse told me it was Mum's favourite spot and that's where she liked to sit and comment on what was going on. He told me that she had been quite 'Catty' about some the workers and residents. They seemed to accept this as part and parcel of the dementia package and they found it quietly amusing. I thought that Mum being rude about the workers was strangely reassuring as it was a sign of the old Mum before she had switched off and had become placid. We took Bowie in to see Mum. When she saw him her face lit up with happiness and he rushed towards her for one of his long cuddles and tickles. It was a great reunion.

'Oh I have missed you Bow'

Then she turned to me and asked where everyone was.

'They have dumped me here!'

She didn't seem to recognise me as the person who had 'dumped' her in the nursing home. I do think she knew I was her daughter, though, it was hard to understand what Mum did and didn't recognise or how aware she was of her situation..

'No one has dumped you in here Mum, this is where you have come to live now, let's go to have a look at your room'

We all walked back to where Mum's room was and someone offered to get us a tray of tea and biscuits. Very civilised I thought.

I took Mum into her bathroom and that's when I noticed that her false teeth were very dirty and seemed to have something stuck on them.

'Let's clean those teeth Mum'

When I went to get her denture pot it was bone dry and the toothpaste was unopened with the cap still covering the end of the toothpaste. The carers obviously hadn't helped Mum or prompted her to brush and clean her teeth. Oh no, I thought this is not good. I do pride myself with high standards as a nurse but this was just basic care. This filled me with anxiety and led to me questioning what help was Mum receiving. The next thing I noticed was that all of her prescribed incontinence pads had been used. There was at least a month's supply of pads and there is no way that Mum would have used them in one week. It was obvious that these had been given to other residents. I never wanted to be that complaining relative that the carers tried to avoid and dreaded coming in, however, something had to be said. I didn't want me complaining to affect the way that the carers treated Mum either. Mum was paying £1600.00 per week for nursing care, this was more costly because of special needs due to her dementia and they weren't even getting the basic care right. I spoke to one of the lovely Care Assistants who I had seen before when Mum was in for respite and to give her due respect, she did appear to be quite horrified herself. She told me that one of the problems was that the nursing home was relying on agency staff to fulfil their resident to staff ratio and she thought that their standards weren't as high as the regular staffs. I asked to speak to the matron and informed her that I was not happy about Mum not having her teeth cleaned since the time I had moved her into the nursing home. I also told her about the amount of incontinence products that had been used which were prescribed and belonged to Mum. I told her that I thought it was disgraceful that these had been given to other residents. Taking these were akin to theft and surely the nursing home had its own supply, otherwise what were these people paying for. To be fair she looked very shocked and told me that she thought it was the agency care staff that had been working there that week that had been looking after Mum. I had not been told that the nursing home was running on mainly agency staff as I thought that they had their own staff. She told me she was sorry about Mum's teeth and the misuse of the pads and assured me that it would not happen again. She told me that they were recruiting for their own staff. The matron told me that she would put corrective action in place immediately, she would make sure that Mum's teeth were cleaned daily and that they would replace the pads. Although, the matron was saying the right things, I didn't quite believe her integrity and wondered whether she was just trying to pacify me. She didn't look me in the eye, her eyes portrayed that she needed to appease the situation. I was left feeling underconfident that Mum's basic care needs would improve. I would need to keep a close eye on the standards of care. This is something that I did not want to do, I just wanted to feel that Mum was in good hands. This poor care started to send my imagination into overdrive, what if they weren't changing her incontinence pads or what if they weren't making sure she is clean after going to the toilet. I started to get a bad feeling about this place which was a shame as it initially appeared to be so promising.

On our visit, Bowie had a lovely time, Andrew took him to see a few other residents. Facial expressions can tell you a lot about what a person is thinking or is feeling. These non-verbal clues are particularly important when a person suffers from dementia, they can tell you if the person is scared, excited or in pain. Quite often a person with dementia may have a facial expression that is blank as if they aren't really there. Sometimes visual expressions are noted and form part of the diagnostic picture. There was one man in the nursing home who suddenly came alive when he saw Bowie. One minute his expression was lifeless and then his expression suddenly changed, he had a big smile and a cheery looking face. The man fussed Bowie and told us how he loved dogs. Bowie lapped up all of the attention. There was another lady who was lying in a recliner chair who appeared to be completely unresponsive and you would even describe her as being in a catatonic state. At first she didn't notice Bowie and then you could see her gradually recognising that there was a dog in the lounge. Suddenly, she sat up and beckoned him over. It was like watching a miracle occurring, she just came to life, stroking Bowie and praising him. In September 2019, Klimova, Toman and Kuca conducted a systematic review of Animal assisted Therapy and in particular the effect that dogs have on patients suffering from Alzheimers disease. They found that dogs can help with improving dementia patients well-being by increasing people's activity levels, reducing agitation, restlessness, disorientation and aggressive behaviour. Dogs can also improve memory and cognition as well as reducing loneliness. Of course we already knew this because we had observed Mum and Bowie. Bowie had taken to Mum immediately when he was a puppy, he acted like her carer, they were always together and he barked at her when she became aggressive which instantly stopped this bad behaviour. Taking Bowie to the nursing home just confirmed what we already suspected, people with dementia benefit from pet therapy.

My next visit to see Mum was equally as disappointing and caused me to have second thoughts about my decision to move her to a nursing home. Now I am not knocking all nursing homes and indeed I have been a manager of a nursing home so I know how good they can be. But first and foremost, before the afternoon teas are offered, the care must be good. In order to achieve this good or excellent care, the right personalities need to be present in the care assistants and there has to be good leadership. It's also not too difficult or demanding to make sure that a person is washed, dressed appropriately, that they have their eyes, teeth and hair cared for. These are basic care needs and do not require specialist skills such as what you expect to find in nursing staff. In order to achieve this standard, the carers need appropriate training and they need to be passionate about care, it's as simple as that. Afterall, we care for ourselves or our children and the principles are the same. I was aware that my expectations were high because that is what I expect of myself. On this occasion and only a few days after the teeth incident, I found Mum sitting in the communal lounge with other residents. The lounge was tastefully decorated in pastel colours and there was a half-circle of chairs in front of the television. The television was on and they looked like they were all watching it but it was an inappropriate program which was not suitable for a group of dementia residents and I could tell that they weren't really interested in it but there was no conversation either. When I spoke to her I realised that she could not hear me. I looked at her ears and it's no wonder she couldn't hear me because she was not wearing her hearing aids. Mum was profoundly deaf without her hearing aids in. This deafness was caused in her younger years when she worked in a noisy sewing mill, at Conlowes in Congleton.

'Where are you hearing aids?' I shouted

'What are you saying?'

I left her in the lounge whilst I went back to her room to look for them. I found them on the side table beside her bed. I took them back to her and pushed them into place into her earlobes. She could then instantly hear me and the television. Again, I felt disappointed as hearing is essential and making sure that she was wearing her hearing aids was just a basic need, surely the person that helped Mum could understand that she needs to hear. One of the batteries had gone flat and the caring staff did not know how to change the battery so I showed them. I kept thinking £1600.00 per week and they don't seem to know the basics. I explained to the nurse in charge that it was very important for Mum to wear her hearing aids, otherwise she would become more isolated which in turn would exacerbate her dementia. The nurse told me that they would write this in her care plan and make sure everyone knew that she must wear the hearing aids. However, on my next visit both hearing aids were missing again and Mum could not hear anything. I felt exasperated, this was causing me distress, why couldn't they get this simple thing right at £1600.00 and where was the leadership? I went to find the nursing home manager who informed me that both hearing aids had been put in the laundry by accident and that they were both broken. I asked her, why I had not been informed but the answer was vague and she didn't seem to be very interested. I asked if the nursing home had an audiologist that visited and they told me that it was something that they were looking in to but they hadn't managed to do this yet because the home was so new. Something had to be done though, I couldn't leave Mum in a world of silence so I decided to take matters in to my own hands.

I phoned Specsavers in Congleton who had an audiologist visit several times a month. Luckily the audiologist was there the following day and they managed to fit us in to the diary once I had explained the urgency of what had happened. I arranged to pick up Mum in the car the following day to take her to the appointment. I asked if the care staff could make sure that Mum was ready to go and well-padded up as I was unaware of anywhere that I would be able to take Mum to change her if she had an accident. Specsavers did have a downstairs disabled toilet but they told me that this was currently being used as a Covid PPE storage area, so Mum would not be able to use this toilet. It is not until you push someone around in a wheelchair that you realise the challenges that they face every day, this includes steps, road curbs, lack of toilet facilities and general access. I left work and went to pick up Mum, they were good to their word and she was ready to leave. I struggled but managed to get Mum into the car and off we went to Congleton. Just as we were driving into Congleton, Mum announced that she needed the toilet. You can't say to someone well there aren't any so you will just have to wee in your pants. Specsavers had told me that I couldn't use their disabled toilet so what was I going to do and then I remembered Morrisons had a disabled toilet. I just prayed that it was accessible and not full of Covid paraphernalia. So we nipped into Morrisons to buy something and to use their disabled toilet. I don't know what disabled people would do if these supermarkets did not provide customer toilets because there aren't many public toilets around these days. The audiologist in Specsavers is a lovely person, always very kind and caring and she remembered Mum. Mum had to have new moulds fitted to her ears and new hearing aids. She had to wait a week for these but I didn't have to take Mum back again, I could just collect the hearing aids when they were ready. So I got Mum back into the car and took her back to the nursing home. I was so tempted to take her home with me but

I didn't. Mum had to be deaf for a week until her new hearing aids arrived. This meant that Mum couldn't hear her visitors, other residents or any of the care staff which meant she was totally isolated which made her more detached. This was due to carelessness but I tried to convince myself that accidents happen and no one meant to wash the hearing aids. I could have cried though, I had managed Mum's care and I had never broken her hearing aids. Communication is so important and even more so when your world is one of total confusion and chaos. A week later on 28th September 2021, I took the new aids to Mum and she could hear again.

I thought and hoped that things may improve now as I was definitely getting a reputation of the annoying visitor. I could see the care staff stiffen when I came to visit. I could imagine my Dad shouting,

'Stand by your beds, Matron is here!'

I never wanted to be the irritating daughter who visits and complains, I wanted to visit Mum and feel like I was part of the team or family. Mum had been there for approximately six weeks and I was hoping for improvement. Allister went to visit Mum one day and he was told that a confused man had got into bed with Mum and this had scared and unsettled her. I was not too concerned with this as that is what happens on dementia wards where people who are confused wander around. It is important to try to maintain people's independence and you can't and should not restrict people. However, I was getting sick of the unavoidable mistakes such as losing Mum's clothes in the laundry, shrinking her jumpers and the lack of basic care. Mum was not getting a shower once a week unless the nice lady carer was working. She continued not to have her hearing aids in or her teeth cleaned. The lack of basic care plus the expense of paying £1600.00 per week for such a poor service was beginning to annoy me. The nursing home continued to rely on filling the staff shortage, particularly at night with agency staff. Some agency staff are good and I know this because I have worked with agency staff and I had also worked as an agency nurse for a while. However, the agency staff cannot know the patients like regular staff and they don't build a rapport with the patients, there is also a lack of continuity which is especially important for people with dementia. I was beginning to have second thoughts about this place. I didn't want to keep moving Mum as that would not be good for her but I seriously needed to consider whether this was the right place for her and I just wanted to take her home with me on every visit. As a nurse, I even offered to do some training on basic care for their staff and free of charge but the nursing home manager said that this would not be allowed and all training was conducted internally. Well train them then, I wanted to shout, train them, lead by example! Allister seemed happier with Mum being there than I was as it was a lot closer to where he lives and worked but he didn't see the lack of care like I did. He wasn't trained like I was and he hadn't cared for Mum like I had. I suppose that it is the downside of knowing too much. I was considering whether there was a way that I could have Mum back at home with me or whether I should consider moving her. The conundrum of having Mum at home, not being able to afford to stop work myself and finding help within Mum's budget was too difficult for me to work out. I held Power of Attorney for both Health and Finances so it was really down to me but it was not a discission to be taken lightly. I was aware that I was not enjoying the lack of control, I had been used to being the number one carer for Mum and now it was out of my control.

⸺◄❖►⸺

Chapter 20

No Time to Say Goodbye

Two days later, on Thursday 30ᵗʰ September, I was at work when I received a phone call in the afternoon asking me to come into the nursing home immediately because Mum was unwell. The nursing home informed me that they had called the paramedics, who were on their way. I rushed over to the nursing home in Willaston which was only a 20 minute drive from work. On arrival I found Mum in her room, sitting in her chair, swaddled in layers and layers of blankets. She looked really poorly and very hot. The staff nurse in charge that afternoon came into Mum's room and told me that she had become unwell in the morning and that they had been observing her all day. The staff nurse told me that when she had come on duty at 2pm, Mum had took a turn for the worse, she had become unresponsive and that is when the paramedics and myself were called. I asked if anyone had called a doctor to see Mum. She told me that the earlier shift hadn't but when she came on duty she immediately knew that Mum needed urgent care and so she had phoned 999. The paramedics had not arrived yet.

I asked if anyone had checked Mum's temperature because she looked like she was boiling up. The staff nurse said that she had checked it and it was only 35.5 degrees centigrade. A normal temperature for a human is around 36 to 37 degrees centigrade. I told the staff nurse that I didn't think that the temperature was accurate because if it was, Mum would be suffering from hypothermia. I asked her to check

Mum's temperature again. I could not believe my eyes, the staff nurse produced one of those totally inaccurate and non-scientific based thermometers that you point at someone's forehead. These became very popular for checking people's temperatures during Covid before entering shops or public places but were totally inaccurate. I asked if she could get an ear thermometer or a real thermometer but she told me that they didn't have one.

'What? You don't have a proper thermometer in the whole of the nursing home?'

'No, we don't'

I was astounded and couldn't believe my ears. I couldn't help myself but to say,

'Surely a nursing home should have a proper and accurate thermometer rather than a gimmick one'.

Just as I was saying this and trying to calm down, two female paramedics arrived and entered Mum's room. They looked at Mum and immediately took off the layers of blankets. They took Mum's temperature with a real thermometer. Mum's temperature was really high at 39.5 degrees centigrade. This was so distressing for me, I thought that Mum was in the care of professional people and they couldn't even recognise that Mum was boiling up. But at least this staff nurse had called the paramedics and had actually managed to get them to attend. However, her temperature was dangerously high and the blankets had been causing her temperature to rise. One of the paramedics then asked why none of the nurses were taking the precaution of wearing PPE as Mum may well have Covid. The paramedics were very concerned about Mum having a severe chest infection or pneumonia and they believed that she needed to be admitted to hospital. They started to prep her for a journey into Leighton hospital. At this point, I panicked,

I said that I didn't want Mum to go into hospital as I thought I would never see her again. All sorts of things were going on in my head, on the one hand, I thought the care would be better in the hospital but on the other hand, she may never get out, particularly if she had Covid. I had the Power of Attorney for her health and wellbeing so I could make the decision not to allow her to go into hospital, If I wished to. I was so torn, I didn't know what to do for the best and then burst into tears. I phoned Allister to ask his opinion but he wasn't really able to comment as he was not there and could not witness how poorly she was. The paramedics were lovely and patient with me, they asked me what I wanted to do. I asked one of them,

'What would you do if it was your Mum?'

'Look this is curable, if this was my Mum I would let her go to hospital for treatment as what she has is an infection which is treatable with IV antibiotics.'

She told me that the hospital were dealing with the Covid isolation better now and that they had a good system. She was very reassuring and so it was decided that they would take Mum to Leighton hospital's A&E unit and I would follow and meet them there. I was allowed to go into the A&E unit at the hospital with Mum because of her Alzheimer's as she would need an advocate and someone who knew her history.

Mum was taken on a blue light to Leighton hospital's A&E unit and I met her there. I had packed a few things for her that I knew she would need such as toiletries, night dresses and tissues. We were allocated a slot in the A&E department, the nurses came to see Mum and took blood, did a Covid test and performed various other tests. I sat with Mum as she drifted in and out of sleep and consciousness. I just sat there next to her in a plastic chair holding her hand and worrying. At least I was with her now but I kept thinking of all the 'What Ifs'. 'What Ifs' can be very damaging and they kept ruminating inside my head. What if she hadn't gone to the nursing home? Would she be poorly now? What if I had just told them it wasn't working out and I had taken her back home and then found a way to care for her myself at home? However, I couldn't just give up work or we wouldn't be able to afford the mortgage.

I sat there for hours and being with Mum was comforting. Mum would come around occasionally, when she woke up to tell me to go home and to get myself off to bed, she seemed to know where she was and appeared to be lucid and really content and comfortable. It's strange how her brain could drift in and out of lucid and confusion so quickly. Approximately, six hours after arriving at the hospital, a doctor came to speak with us. The doctor told us that Mum was free of Covid which was a relief, however; she did had pneumonia and she needed to be admitted for intravenous fluids and antibiotics. The doctor said she was very dehydrated which may have been a causable factor. I was asked to sign a Do Not Resuscitate form known as a DNR form. I informed the doctor that I held power of attorney for her health and wellbeing and if they were to make any decisions on her care, please could they call me. This was written on her notes. Although I was allowed to be with Mum in A&E, I was not allowed onto the ward. There was a strict no visiting rule in place due to Covid, however, they had a system in place that a designated nurse would call the next of kin every morning with an update. This process was to stop the phone lines being jammed with incoming calls. So I said my goodbyes to Mum in the corridor, told her that I loved her, kissed her on the cheek and off she went. I let Allister know that Mum was being admitted and then I drove home which took an hour, I got home at 1am and managed to sleep despite my brain being very busy ruminating. I was worried sick and wondering if Mum would ever leave the hospital. I was remembering during the first wave of Covid, that visitors were not allowed to see their loved ones even when they were dying. It was a terrible period of time for close relatives when their loved ones were admitted to hospital and the after effects of this enforced separation are still impacting people's mental health now. Only this time, it was us, we were not allowed to visit Mum. I was so concerned that she may think we didn't care about her.

The hospital were good to their word and at 11am I received a phone call from Mum's designated nurse. The nurse informed me that Mum had been peaceful during the night and was comfortable. She had woken up and had a drink and her temperature had reduced with the intravenous antibiotics and saline drip. For the next few days I would wait for my phone call at 11 am which were both reassuring and pleasing as it seemed that Mum was responding well to the treatment plan. By day four and five, Mum had been out of bed and was entertaining the nurses and seemed to be enjoying the experience of being in hospital I was told. When the nurse spoke to me she asked,

'Are you Isabel?'

'Yes that's me.'

'Well we have heard a lot about you! She has been telling us all that you are a matron.'

'That is what my parents have always called me, I am not a matron now but I am a registered nurse.'

'Well she is very proud of you.'

She had been commenting on the cleaning staff and saying how she used to be a Caretaker and that her daughter was a nursing matron. She had been keeping the nurses and care assistants on their toes, telling them that I would be inspecting their work. It was great to hear that she was in good spirits. The nurses told me they were surprised of how well she was doing, considering how poorly she was initially. I think she had even been a little critical of their work ethics which amused them and it showed me that she was actually on the mend. It was likely that she would be discharged soon and I needed to make some important decisions. Should I let Mum go back to the nursing home where they didn't seem to know how to take a residents temperature, did not have basic clinical equipment such as a thermometer, where they lost her clothes, broke her hearing aid and didn't seem to help her with her daily activities of living?

To be quite honest I was less than impressed with the lack of basic care at the nursing home. Some of the staff were amazing and lovely but there were not enough of them. Some of the carers just seemed like they were there because it was a job, they didn't seem to be passionate about care. Providing cream teas for relatives is great but only if the care is good. There were too many agency staff being used at the nursing home to make the it feel like a family and a home. I was having serious doubts about my decision to send her there in the first place and I just wanted to bring her back home. The nursing home did look like a hotel and staff always offered you a drink and biscuit when you were visiting but to me that is not what is important. The nursing home did not seem as good as it was when Mum went there for respite care. I wanted to believe that when I was not there, Mum was getting total holistic care. There is no excuse for lack of basic care. Dentures, teeth, hair and nails should all be part of the daily care plan. The care plan should not be a document that is produced to prove you have one, it should be a working document which should be available to all nursing and care staff. Then there was the hearing aid issue, it's not difficult to make sure that the patient has their hearing aid in. This is particularly important for a nursing home which has residents with dementia because they need to preserve and promote communication as effectively as possible. I needed to decide what to do next but I was also aware that a routine and familiarity were essential for Mum too. It was one of the hardest decisions I have ever made for Mum to go into a nursing home in the first place with so much disruption to Mum's life. How could I upturn her life again?

On day seven of her hospital stay which was Thursday 7th October, I got the usual phone call at 11 am but the nurse told me that Mum was not as alert today and that she was very sleepy and a little unresponsive. The nurse told me that it was nothing to worry about but she was going to get the doctor to check her over later that day. I did worry though all day, how could I not worry. However, I was very happy with the care and treatment that they had given to Mum so far and I needed to trust the staff. That same day I had started with a heavy cold myself and didn't feel too well. The following morning was strange because I didn't receive the expected phone call. I was really worried because the day before Mum had not been well. I left it until midday and then I thought no I can't sit around waiting, especially because the nurse had told me that Mum was poorly the day before. I decided to phone the ward myself rather than wait any longer. I telephoned the hospital switch board and got transferred directly to the ward. After several rings the ward clark answered and I told her that I was enquiring about Mrs Sybil Boote, who was my Mum and that I was concerned as no one had phoned me. She told me that she would get the nursing sister. I waited for a few minutes and started to worry that something was very wrong. The nursing sister came to the phone and I confirmed who I was and that I was next of kin to Mrs Sybil Boote and that I wanted to know if she was any better as she was unwell the day before plus I was phoning because I hadn't received my usual phone call from her designated nurse.

'Mrs Boote has gone.'

I couldn't hide the sarcasm and horror in my voice.

'Do you mean she has died or do you mean that she has been discharged?'

'I mean Mrs Boote was discharged this morning back to the nursing home.'

'I was not informed of this and I may not have wanted her to go back to the nursing home, I may have wanted her to come home to me. I do have power of attorney for her health, it was written in her notes to phone me before any decisions were made. You should have consulted me before discharging her!'

'I'm really sorry, you are right someone should have called you, she had already left when I came on duty. I am so sorry!'

'I appreciate that you are all busy but this is my Mum and someone should have called me. We can't go back in time though so please make sure your staff know that they were out of order, not to call her next of kin'.

'I will do, and I am sorry'

'I was told that she was poorly yesterday so why would they discharge her today'

'I don't know, I'm sorry, she must have been discharged after the doctors round this morning before I came on shift'.

I was distraught. I ended the call and phoned the nursing home. The staff on duty at the nursing home said that Mum had just returned in an ambulance.

'She just arrived unannounced in an ambulance. We thought you must have known but no one informed us of her discharge.'

'No, I had no idea that they were discharging her, especially as they told me she was very poorly yesterday. How is she, anyway?'

The staff nurse told me that Mum seems alright and that she had even managed to walk out of the ambulance and was pleased to be back. She told me that when Mum came back the first thing that she had said was,

'Oh, am I so glad to be back'

I thanked the nurse on the telephone and asked her to tell Mum that Allister would come to see her tomorrow and that I would be coming to see her on the Sunday. Sunday would be 10th October 2021. I had a heavy cold and didn't want to give that to her as she was just recovering from pneumonia so I thought I would leave visiting her for a day. I was so angry with the hospital for not consulting with me or for at least telling me that she was being discharged. What was the point of the power of attorney for health? Was it just a piece of paper that no one considered? I decided that there was no point making a complaint though either as the hospital had done an amazing job up until that last omission and non-existent communication. Poor communication is the root cause of the majority of complaints in hospitals and yet there is little or no training in this area for staff. There was also no point complaining as the NHS was on its knees, Covid had felled it and I was not going to add to their stress. Also Mum was safe and no real harm had been done I suppose. I phoned Allister to let him know and he said he would visit Mum the next day.

'Give her my love and tell her I will be in to see her on Sunday'

'Will do'

'We will also need to talk about whether Mum should stay there or not but that can wait until she has recuperated'.

The next day, Allister went to see Mum. He phoned me to tell me that Mum was sitting in her chair in her room, she was very sleepy and quiet. She was dressed but she looked very frail. He also told me that he had sat and cried throughout his visit. Mum had drifted in and out of sleep but she was aware of his presence. He stayed for about an hour and then left her to sleep.

That evening Andrew and I went to bed as usual at about 10.30pm. At 2am I received a call from the nursing home. When you get a call in the middle of the night, you instantly know it's not going to be good news. I sat bolt upright in bed and answered the call. My heart was racing and inside I knew it was bad news. It was a male agency staff nurse on the phone to tell me that Mum had died in her sleep. He was very empathetic and spent some time talking to me. I tried to listen to his words but it was difficult to concentrate, my throat and chest were constricting with grief. He patiently explained that he had been doing his rounds and giving out medication at 10pm and he had sat with Mum for about 15 minutes. She was holding his hand and didn't want him to leave her but he needed to go to the other patients so he had settled her down and left her room. I tried to imagine this frightened elderly and poorly lady reaching for his hand and not wanting to let him go. Did she know she was going to die, I wondered? Did she have that feeling of impending doom? He continued to tell me that had gone back to check in on her at 1am and she was dead. He told me that she looked peaceful, he said that there were no signs that she was deteriorating earlier on, when he was with her at 10pm, otherwise he would have called me.

'Did she die alone then?'

'Yes she died in her sleep, she looked peaceful but she was alone'

I asked him who else was on duty to find out if any of the care staff that I knew were on duty so I could speak to them. There wasn't anyone working that I knew and more importantly there were no care staff that Mum would have known either. He told me that there were four agency staff on duty that night. That was terrible, just horrible to think that Mum died alone and to realise that before she died when she was holding onto the hand of the nurse in charge, not wanting to be left alone, no one was there to comfort her. He told me that the doctor had been in to certify her death at 1am on 10th October 2021. He told me that I could visit Mum if I wanted to or she could go to the funeral directors directly. I ended the call, distraught, inconsolable, choked with sadness and regret.

'Mum's dead, she died alone' I told Andrew through body wrenching sobs. He put his arms around me in a comforting embrace and held me.

'I need to let Allister know.'

'Do you want me to call him?'

'No it should be me.'

I phoned Allister and told him. He didn't seem surprised as he had seen how frail and poorly she was the day before. He told me that he didn't want to go to view her body as he wanted to remember her the way she was. In my state of shock, at 2am I also phoned the undertaken and bless her she answered the phone and she was so lovely with me even though I was disturbing her in the middle of the night. She persuaded me to go to see Mum in the nursing home as she thought it would be nicer for me to see her in her bed rather than at the morgue. I am glad she did persuade me to go to see Mum as the nursing home had made Mum look nice. I spent some time with Mum and apologised to her for letting her down, for not being with her when she was dying, for not keeping her safe at home. The worst part for me was that I never said goodbye to her, the last time I had seen her was ten days before when she was taken away from me in A&E to go to the ward. The thought of her dying and being totally alone is something that I thought was both heartbreaking and devastating. I have a strong belief that people should not die alone or in pain if it can be prevented. If I had know she had so little time on this earth I would have nursed her at home just as I had done for Dad. I was devastated and I had a building feeling of guilt that I couldn't shake off.

I stayed with Mum for about half an hour. However, her soul had already left her body and just an empty shell was left. I went to the nurse in charge and told them that I was leaving. They said they were sorry for my loss. They also told me I had a week to remove Mum's belongs.

Chapter 21

Aftermath

The next day was full of phone calls to let everyone know that Mum had died. I got Mum's phone book and systematically worked my way through it, starting with family and then moving on to friends. I let Mum's carers know who looked after her when she was at home. Sharon, Karen and Debbie were really upset as I knew they would be. That week was consumed with the practicalities required following the death of a loved one. There was so much to do, such as arranging the funeral, speaking to the vicar for the church, organising the burial and getting the headstone removed from Dad's grave so that Mum could be reunited with him in death. I had to go back to the nursing home to collect Mum's things, this was very upsetting. I arrived at the nursing home and they had kindly packed things up, they had locked her room so that no other dementia patients could mess with Mum's things. On top of her walker was a bag and on top of that sat Mum's blue hat. Her beloved blue sunhat. I thanked the staff in the British polite way you do, even though you are not that happy and left quietly. Next was the death certificate which needed to be registered. You used to have to take the death certificate to the registry office but now it can be done online. You have to let lots of agencies know about a death, such as social services but luckily they have a form now called 'Tell us Once' which informs many of the agencies in one go. Then there is the finances which needed to be frozen, apart from the funeral money which the bank can pay directly to the undertakers.

The things you have to do and you are supposed to know how to do, at a time when functioning is difficult because of grief are huge. Luckily, the undertakers were there to guide and steer us along. There is so much to do leading up to the funeral and beyond that there is no time to grieve. You need to pick a coffin, do you go for solid oak or wicker which is more environmentally friendly? Mum was getting buried and placed on top of Dad so we opted for Oak. Allister had a special piece of Oak that he wanted to place in-between Mum and Dad so that had to be discussed with the undertakers and the grave diggers. What flowers did we want? What hymns , if any? What would Mum wear? Embalming or not embalming? Who was to carry the coffin? These were just a few of the choices that we needed to make. I had to make sure that there was disabled access for my Uncle George to get into the church as he insisted on saying his goodbyes to his sister. After the funeral, we were hiring the village hall so that people could have refreshments. We had to choose what food and drink we wanted and we needed to let the caters know how many people would be attending. This was really difficult to guess as it is not the same as a wedding where people RSVP. It was important to try to get this just right for Mum, just like she had in the past. It's a strange feeling if you are the one doing all of the arrangements as you have to compartmentalise your grief and the tasks that you need to achieve. Therefore for anyone observing you, it looks like you are taking everything in your stride and that grief has been bypassed. I looked like I was processing everything with ease but inside I was tormented and traumatised by the loss of Mum. I could not get past that she had died alone and that I had let her down. Why couldn't I have kept her with me, safe?

The funeral day arrived and everything was in place. Mum was ready to join Dad forever. Our house was miles away from the church so we arranged for the funeral procession to go from Allister's house. Mum was to be joining Dad who was buried in the church yard at All Saints Church, Church Lawton. All Saints Church is very old, quaint and welcoming. It is a very small church with a tower and it dates back to the 11th Century although it is not completely original as there was a fire in 1798 which destroyed the main building but it was rebuilt in 1803 in a Neo-classical style in brick. The tower is older dating back to the 16th century in sandstone. The church is perched on top of an incline and the path to access the huge church doors was steep. The grave yard has a very uneven path circling around the back of the church, crooked old grave stones line each side of the path. The church yard is immaculately kept, serene and overlooks farmland which gives a feel of tranquillity. Mum and Dad were always impressed by neatness and they were always saying what a tidy church this was. Dad was also impressed with the soil. He would tell me how it drains well which means that the coffins stay dry. I was never too keen on this conversation but Dad would just continue on. He was quite right really, death is the only certainty that we know. Dying of natural causes means that the cause is internal rather than an external cause such as a trauma. Dying is part and parcel of living and we cannot avoid it. Dad wanted to be cremated but Mum persuaded him to be buried so that she could join him. I thought well he must love her as he knew he was going first but agreed to be buried so that she knew that she would not be alone in the soil. Dad had said to me just before he died 'well at least they won't have to worry about my pacemaker blowing up in the furnace, there is a pile of them at the Crem.' He also informed me that the services are pushed through quickly at the Crem because there is always the next one coming in behind but with a burial there is no rush. How he knew this stuff I don't know but he was always practical and he was never afraid of the inevitable.

We were driven in the funeral car to the church, Andrew had followed in our car so that we weren't stranded at the church once the service and burial was over. The church was full with friends and family, there weren't quite as many people there as there was for Dad's funeral. For his funeral, there were so many people there, people couldn't sit down and they had to stand at the back of the church. Quite a few of their friends and some family had also died in the five years since Dad had left us. As we walked down the aisle to the front pews, I could feel eyes following us. Sympathy hung heavy in the air. Mum's coffin was placed on a stand at the front of the church with her blue straw hat sat on top. Mum's funeral was conducted by a pleasant and modern female vicar. I had picked Mum's favourite hymns, All things bright and beautiful and Abide with me. Mum was quite religious but she never really attended church on a weekly basis but she was a believer. Prayers were read and then in the middle of the service, the vicar said a few words about Mum. She talked about Mum's grandchildren who had all contributed to the eulogy. What the vicar did do bizarrely was to use my name instead of Mum's. She proceeded to say,

'Today we lay to rest, Isabel. We are here to celebrate the beautiful life you lived and the love you shared."

Allister coughed, the congregation shuffled uncomfortably but she didn't noticed.

'Isabel's friends and family gather today to show their respects.'

Someone muted 'Sybil'. I heard someone giggle behind me.

'Isabel will join Alan.'

I started thinking, 'Bloody Hell' it's like I am at my own funeral. This is like looking into the future, this will be what it's like. I couldn't move or say anything to correct her, the shock and grief had me rendered useless. Also, what was a supposed to say? It's not me! It was the most surreal experience of my life, one that is was not too happy about at the time but one that I have laughed about since. There was also part of me that wanted to burst into hysterical laughter. This went on and the vicar didn't seem to get the hints that were being aimed at her quite vocally now. We are very English though and we didn't want to interrupt the vicar so on it went until someone from the side spoke up.

'Sybil! It's Sybil, not Isabel'

Following the funeral we went over to the village hall for refreshments and to chat with our close friends and family. Of course, the talk was about Mum but also of the bizarre events in the church. Gradually the hall emptied and life carried on. We all hugged each other and said goodbye. Andrew drove us home feeling empty and bereft. I felt slightly flu like as you do following prolonged crying. Bowie was waiting for us and he looked forlorn. Could he sense the loss?

Then once the funeral had past, there are other things that need to be done such as the probate form to complete. I had already had a bit of practice with these probate forms. I had arranged the funeral and the probate on behalf of Aunty Pam when Uncle Sam died. Then there was my Dad's funeral and Probate form in the same year so I was becoming quite efficient at this. What a thing to say you are good at. So, I followed the same routine for Mum's funeral taking in her wishes. The probate forms following Mum's death were more tricky because the money wasn't automatically going to her spouse. Completing the probate form and attachments for Mum's estate was requiring the skills of an accountant. The

Estate is a strange word to use as it conjures up an image of a mansion, masses of land and grandeur. In reality Mum had very little in the way of money or valuables but everything has to be accounted for. I can understand why lots of people give this job to a solicitor but I did manage to work my way through it.

Once all of the practicalities are over, you have more time to reflect on everything. For me these reflects could occur at any time, they would creep up on me and very unannounced. It could happen when I was driving and I started thinking about Mum or Dad or both of them. It could happen in the middle of the night whilst Andrew was sleeping soundly next to me. These judgements would just appear and overtake any other thoughts. My judgements and thoughts are always around regret and I can list them:

- I regret taking Mum into a nursing home. I shouldn't have done this. I am therefore, a bad person, a bad daughter.

- I regret not going to see Mum the day she got out of hospital even though I had a heavy cold. I should have gone to see her. She would have thought that I didn't care for her. I am therefore, a bad person, a bad daughter.

- I regret that I was not strong enough to manage with Mum at home. Why was I weak, so what if I couldn't go to work, what was more important. I put work before Mum, therefore I am a bad person and a bad daughter. I let her down.

- I regret not researching the staffing levels more and understanding that sometimes the nursing was run purely with agency nurses who would not know Mum. I was dazzled by the new build and convinced myself that it was lovely and therefore the care was good. I should have chosen somewhere else. I should better after all I am a nurse. Why didn't I take Mum out of there when I knew things weren't as good as they looked. I let Mum down.

I would then have terrible visions of Mum being frightened at the end of her life with no one to hold her hand or she would be calling out and no one would hear her. She would be in her room, not coherent enough to know how to use a call bell because of her dementia. Shut in her room, unable to get anyone to hear her calls. The worse vision is Mum dying alone. The guilt I felt and still feel is unbearable at times. People are constantly telling me that I could not have done more and that I did everything I could for Mum. It doesn't matter how many times I am told this, I still bear the guilt and wear it like a badge. It is my belief that I let my Mum down at the very end when she needed me and because of this she died alone and I never said goodbye. I have been left bereft, this is not because I lost Mum, it's because I believe that the loss of Mum was done badly. I know this because when Dad died, he died the way he wanted to in comfort, not alone and without any poor care leading up to his death. This allowed me to move through the grief process easily. Whereas, I am trapped in a whirlpool of self-disappointment and regret.

I have tried to understand why I felt so bereft about Mum's death and tried to look at it from a professional point of view. To do this I looked at the grief process. According to Cruse there are five stages of grief are Deniel, Anger, Bargaining, Depression and Acceptance. They describe grief coming in waves which is exactly what I have experienced with both Dad and Mum. They also say that you can move in and out of the stages which I can recognise in myself. Acceptance came quite quickly for me following Dad's death but I am waiting and hoping for this acceptance following Mum's death.

One of the reasons why I decided to write this book was because I thought it may help me to achieve some acceptance. I thought it may be cathartic. Another reason for writing the book was to share and highlight the pleasures of caring for a relative with dementia and to show how families adapt to extreme situations and circumstances. Without a doubt there have been many comical and entertaining moments throughout this journey. However, there are true challenges for anyone caring for a relative with dementia and this is also true for other family members living in the same house. There needs to be a great deal of understanding from family members who you live with and for Andrew's support I will always be eternally grateful.

There is little or no support following diagnosis of dementia. There is little or no support for family's who decide to take some weight away from the NHS and take on the responsibility of caring for a relative. Cultures have changed over the years and in modern society it is no longer seen as a responsibility of the family to care for a relative with dementia or other aging illness. Another reason why people don't take on the responsibility of caring for a elderly person especially one with dementia is that they just can't afford to give up work to care for a relative full time. Again, culture has changed and gone are the days when the female family member could or would want to stay at home to care for children and elderly relatives, especially now that most households rely on two wages. The means test for support is brutal. Carers allowance is only available if the elderly person is claiming a qualifying benefit and also if the carer Is earning a low wage. The carer allowance is low which does not make it financially viable for a person to give up work to become a full time care giver. There are very few incentives for caring for an elderly relative other than love. Unfortunately, love does not pay the mortgage and other bills though which often leaves the relatives trying to find a way to work and at the same time be a carer. Maybe if there were incentives for caring for an elderly relative at the relatives home there may be more people willing to do this and there would be less requirements on the NHS thus saving the government money as well as freeing up precious hospital beds.

The money that the elderly person has needs to be carefully managed and rationed in order to last them for the rest of their lives. This financial pressures of caring for an elderly relative can lead to further demands on the care giver. High demands and no control are the perfect recipe for stress. The lack of control is more damaging than high pressure. The relatives of people suffering from dementia take on a huge and challenging responsibility through love and devotion to a loved one. By doing this they save the NHS and government a lot of money. In my opinion there should be a more support available to these people, maybe just a few hours of free care per week similar to that of nursery placements. We should all be concerned about this because as is well documented, the population is becoming older, people are living for longer and at the same time there are less hospital beds. The latest statistics estimates that one in three people will develop dementia in their old age. The old peripheral hospitals have long closed and so this is a growing crisis. Surely it would be beneficial to support families trying to care for their own relatives in their own home. The relatives are not trying to preserve any money for their own inheritance, they are trying to ration the money so that it will last. In some ways it could be argued that the way the system works is that it is more beneficial to an elderly person to have very little money. Anyone with more than £23,250 has to self-fund all care, if they have less money than that sum, then the government contribute towards the care. Mum had to self-fund because of her house sale, she was paying £1600 per week to the nursing home for care that did not meet her basic needs. I estimated that Mum could live there for about a year and then I had no idea what would happen next. This was a great worry to me and I didn't know if I would have to move Mum. The government website states that the government will pay a flat rate of £209.19 towards nursing home care but what would that mean once Mum had less than £23,250. No one seemed to be able to provide an answer. This was also compounded by the lack of places willing to take elderly people with Alzheimers and dementia care is more expensive than general nursing care.

We should also care about the training provided in private nursing homes. There is the Care Quality Commission (CQC) scheme which will provide a rating of poor to excellent. The nursing home that I chose for Mum had a Good rating and it did indeed look lovely, some of the staff were fantastic and when Mum went in there for respite care whilst we went on holiday for a week the care appeared to be good. However, when she had gone into the nursing home for respite care there were only a handful of residents as the nursing home had only just opened. In my opinion, the nursing home care was let down by not having a sufficient ratio of regular staff and there was obviously a lack of staff training in basic care. The CQC is a snap shot of care at the time of the assessment. At the nursing home, sometimes the care was good but when Mum moved in a permanent resident there was certainly room for major improvement. The nursing home was new which may have been a factor as they were not fully staffed and relied heavily on agency staff. I do not have a problem with agency staff as they are needed to fill in for sickness and holidays but there should never be a full quota of agency staff running a nursing home because they are not familiar with the clinical policies and procedures or the emergency procedures but most importantly they don't know the residents. The night of my Mum's death, there were no permanent nursing home staff working which I found distressing because they didn't know Mum so they would not have recognised a deterioration or understood her needs.

The end of life process is crucially important to the person as well as to the relatives. When my Dad who had cancer was dying we had the support of Hospice at Home and they were fantastic. The support we received for Dad's end of life compared to Mum was world's apart. Dad was cared for whilst Mum was just left to die alone and with no one who knew her on duty. Alzheimer's is not acknowledged or really seen as terminal illness either, which it is! No one recovers from Alzheimer's despite some of the ground breaking research that is happening in this area. I strongly believe that it is not given the same respect or credence of cancer. Dementia is accompanied with a stigma, it is the impoverished relative to other diseases such as cancer. The poor communication on the day of Mum's discharge from the hospital and the willingness to basically throw her out of hospital in order to free up a bed, when I had been told the day before that she was unwell is another major contribution to how Mum's end of life care was done badly. Communication is so important at any time but at the end of life it is paramount. Good communication aids the relatives through the grief process. The last few weeks of Mum's life had like a domino effect which resulted in the process of bereavement being more difficult than it needed to be.

I had started to consider my own destiny. Grandma Beech had Alzheimer's disease and had died of pneumonia, just like my Mum had. The question that keeps entering my conscious mind, is whether this pattern of illness is going to be my future. Alzheimer's is not genetically inherited but the literature says that that you are more likely to get dementia if your parent has. The risk of developing Alzheimer's disease increases the older you get. One in fourteen people over the age of 65 years old and one in every six people will develop Alzheimer's disease. Even more worryingly, one in twenty people will develop Alzheimer's disease before the age of 65 years old. This is call Early-onset Alzheimer's disease according to the NHS. The Alzheimer's Society quote that one in three people will develop dementia in their lifetime. These are frightening statistics. Some research conducted in 2021 states that people who suffer from chronic migraine are more likely to develop Alzheimer's disease particularly in females. I suffer from chronic migraine which can be very debilitating and can cause significant brain fog. Some statistics say that chronic migraine suffers are three times more likely to develop Alzheimer's disease. These statistics are scientific. Knowing what I know, the thought of developing Alzheimer's disease is terrifying. As with Alice, is this my looking glass for the future? Will this mean that I will pass over to the strange parallel world in the twilight zone just like Mum and Grandma Beech? My conclusion is that is highly likely considering the statistics. Therefore, I need to do everything in my power to try to preserve my cognitive functions and I will be on a quest to do so. I do see some positivity in the fact that knowledge is growing on about Alzheimer's disease and brain functioning in general. There are more preventative and effective medicines now available as well as ongoing research which gives me hope for my future. Without hope we have nothing.

••••━━◄◈►━━••••

References

- Alzheimer's Society, Dementia was the leading cause of death in Britain for the last 10 years, accessed on 29th October 2024 from

  https://www.alzheimers.org.uk/about-us/dementia-UK-leading-cause-of-death

- Alzheimer's Society, Facts for the media about dementia, accessed on 29th October 2024 from

  https://www.alzheimers.org.uk/about-us/news-and-media/facts-media

- Kilmova, Toman, Kuca (2019), Effectiveness of the dog therapy for patients with dementia – as systematic review, accessed on 29th October 2024 from

  https://bmcpsychiatry.biomedcentral.com/articles/10.1186/s12888-019-2245-x

- NHS, Overview, Alzheimer's disease, accessed on 29th October 2024 from

  https://www.nhs.uk/conditions/alzheimers-disease/

- Office of National statistics, Coronavirus (Covid-19): 2020 in charts, accessed on 29th October 2024 from

  https://www.ons.gov.uk/peoplepopulationand community/healthandsocialcare/ conditionsanddiseases/ articles/coronaviruscovid192020incharts/2020-12-18

- Office of National statistics, Dementia and Alzheimer's disease deaths including comorbidities, England and Wales: 2019 registrations, accessed on 29th October 2024 from

https://www.ons.gov.uk/
peoplepopulationandcommunity/
birthsdeathsandmarriages/ deaths/ bulletins/
dementiaandalzheimersdiseasedeathsincluding
comorbiditiesenglandandwales/ 2019registrations